Pallavi Ahluwalia
Editor

Ghansham Biyani
Associate Editor

Handbook of Perioperative Analgesia

Springer

Editor
Pallavi Ahluwalia
Department of Anesthesia
Teerthanker Mahaveer Medical College (TMMC)
Moradabad, Uttar Pradesh, India

Associate Editor
Ghansham Biyani
Department of Anesthesiology
All India Institute of Medical Sciences (AIIMS)
Mangalagiri, Andhra Pradesh, India

ISBN 978-981-96-7821-1 ISBN 978-981-96-7822-8 (eBook)
https://doi.org/10.1007/978-981-96-7822-8

This Springer imprint is published by the registered company Springer Nature Singapore Pte Ltd.
The registered company address is: 152 Beach Road, #21-01/04 Gateway East, Singapore 189721, Singapore

*Dedicated to my husband,
Dr. Amit Ahluwalia, my rock,
the unwavering foundation
upon which I built this dream.
And to my wonderful children,
Shaurya and Sharanya, whose
boundless energy and
overflowing love filled every
corner of my world while
I wrote.*

*Thank you for your
unwavering support, for the
countless cups of tea, the quiet
understanding, and for filling
my days with joy, even amidst
the late nights and writer's
block. Your laughter was the
music that kept me going, and
your belief in me, the light
that guided my way.*

Your patience during the moments of distraction, your encouragement when I doubted myself, and your genuine excitement for this project meant more than words can express. This book is a testament to your love and support, a story woven with the threads of our shared life. I dedicate it to you, with all my heart.

Foreword

In the ever-evolving landscape of medical practice, the management of pain, particularly in the perioperative setting, remains a cornerstone of patient care. As surgical techniques advance and anesthesia evolves, the need for effective analgesia has never been more critical. The *Handbook of Perioperative Analgesia* serves as a comprehensive resource for clinicians dedicated to improving patient outcomes through enhanced pain management strategies.

The multidisciplinary approach to perioperative care necessitates a deep understanding of pharmacological interventions, regional anesthesia techniques, and the latest evidence-based practices. Within these pages, you will find a wealth of information that not only covers the foundational concepts of analgesia but also delves into innovative techniques and emerging trends that are shaping the future of perioperative medicine.

The contributors to this textbook are experts in their respective fields, bringing a wealth of knowledge and experience to the forefront. Their insights will guide you through complex decision-making processes, addressing both common and unique challenges faced in various surgical contexts.

The Editor, Dr. Pallavi Ahluwalia, deserves immense praise for curating such a comprehensive and insightful resource. Her meticulous attention to detail and commitment to advancing the field is evident on every page. By bringing together contributions from leading experts, the editor has created a valuable reference that will undoubtedly enhance the knowledge and practices of healthcare professionals. This book stands as a testament to her dedication and expertise in the realm of perioperative care.

Effective perioperative analgesia is not just about reducing pain; it is about enhancing the overall patient experience, minimizing complications, and promoting recovery. By integrating the principles and practices outlined in this book into your daily routine, you will be better equipped to provide compassionate, evidence-based care that prioritizes the well-being of your patients.

May this hand book serve as a valuable resource and inspire a continued commitment to excellence in perioperative analgesia.

Director APMC, AAS Pain Management Centre
Rohtak, Haryana, India
Former Senior Professor & Head, Department of Cardiac Anaesthesia & Pain Management Centre
PGIMS
Rohtak, Haryana, India

Naveen Malhotra

Preface

In the ever-evolving field of medicine, the management of pain, particularly in the perioperative setting, stands as a critical pillar for patient care. The nuances and complexities associated with perioperative analgesia necessitate a comprehensive understanding and meticulous application of various pain management strategies to ensure patient comfort, facilitate recovery, and minimize complications. This textbook, *Handbook of Perioperative Analgesia*, aspires to bridge the gap between foundational knowledge and advanced clinical practice, serving as an indispensable resource for healthcare professionals.

The impetus for this book arose from the recognition of the diverse approaches to pain management that span across different surgical specialties and patient populations. By encompassing a broad spectrum of topics—from the underlying mechanisms of pain to the latest advancements in analgesic techniques—this textbook aims to provide a holistic and integrated perspective on perioperative analgesia. The contributions of leading experts in anesthesiology, surgery, pharmacology, and pain management have been meticulously curated to offer readers an authoritative and up-to-date resource.

Each chapter has been crafted to address both theoretical and practical aspects of perioperative analgesia. Starting with the fundamentals of pain physiology and pharmacology, the text progresses through various analgesic modalities, including systemic medications, regional anesthesia techniques, and multimodal approaches. Special attention is given to patient-specific considerations, such as age, comorbidities, and the type of surgical procedure, ensuring that the information is applicable to a wide array of clinical scenarios.

In addition to traditional pain management strategies, this book delves into emerging therapies and technologies that are shaping the future of perioperative care. Innovations in drug delivery systems, the role of genetic and molecular markers in personalized medicine, and the integration of minimally invasive surgical techniques are explored in depth. By keeping abreast of these advancements, healthcare providers can enhance their clinical acumen and improve patient outcomes.

The *Handbook of Perioperative Analgesia* is designed to serve as a comprehensive reference for medical students, residents, practicing clinicians, and researchers. Whether you are seeking to solidify your understanding of basic principles or explore the cutting-edge developments in perioperative pain management, this book offers valuable insights and practical guidance.

It is with profound gratitude that I acknowledge the invaluable contributions of my esteemed associate editor, Dr. Ghanshyam Biyani, in the creation of this book. His expertise, dedication, and meticulous attention to detail have been instrumental in shaping this comprehensive guide. His collaborative spirit and unwavering commitment have greatly enriched the depth and quality of this work. Dr. Ghanshyam Biyani, thank you for your exceptional support and for being an indispensable part of this journey.

I extend my heartfelt gratitude to the contributors whose expertise and dedication have made this textbook a reality. Their commitment to advancing the field of perioperative analgesia is reflected in the depth and breadth of the content presented herein. I also thank our readers for their pursuit of excellence in patient care, and I hope that this hand book will serve as a trusted companion in your clinical practice and professional development.

Moradabad, Uttar Pradesh, India — Pallavi Ahluwalia

Contents

Editors and Contributors

About the Editors

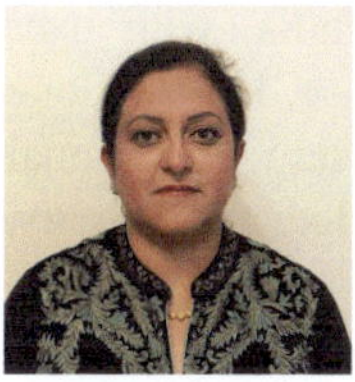

Pallavi Ahluwalia MD, MNAMS, PGDHHM, CEPC, FIMSA, FRCP (Glas.) is presently Senior Professor in the Department of Anesthesiology, Teerthanker Mahaveer Medical College in Moradabad, India, with over 25 years of experience. She is the Ex-Head of Department, Emergency Medicine, Rohilkhand Medical College, Bareilly. Her research focuses on innovative pain relief techniques and enhancing patient outcomes during the perioperative period. She is a fellow of the Royal College of Physicians and Surgeons (Glasgow) and specializes in perioperative analgesia, with additional Fellowship in Palliative medicine from the Institute of Palliative Medicine and St. Christopher's Hospice, London. She is a Fellow of the International Medical Science Academy. She has published many peer-reviewed international publications and has contributed chapters to various issues of the "Yearbook of Anesthesiology." She is President of the Indian Society of Anesthesia, Moradabad branch. She has received several awards, including the IMA

National Award for Excellence in Anesthesia Research and the Annual M.K. Dey Award from the Indian College of Anaesthesia. She is past Editor-in-Chief *Indian Journal of Clinical Anaesthesia*. She is MD and DNB appraiser and examiner. She is an eminent faculty and has organized various conferences and workshops.

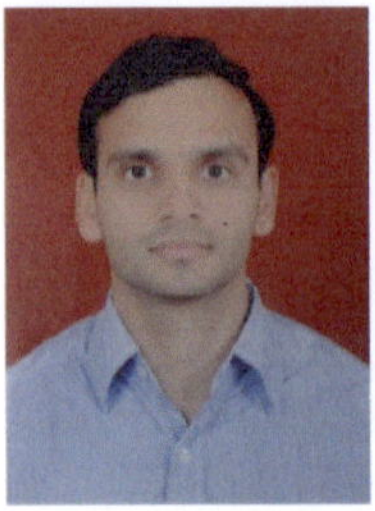

Ghansham Biyani MD, DNB, MNAMS, EDAIC is presently working as Associate Professor in the Department of Anesthesiology at All India Institute of Medical Sciences Mangalagiri, Andhra Pradesh, India, with over 10 years of clinical experience. He has done one year of clinical fellowship in regional anesthesia from Cambridge University, UK. His areas of interest and research include regional and obstetric anesthesia. He is a member of "Cadaveric Research Academic Board" and has organized many workshops on ultrasound-guided regional anesthesia. He has published over 60 peer-reviewed articles in national and international journals and has contributed many chapters in various textbooks on regional anesthesia. He is the section editor of *Journal of Anaesthesiology Clinical Pharmacology* and the *Indian Anaesthetists Forum* journals and has received excellent reviewer award for his contribution.

Contributors

Pallavi Ahluwalia, MD, MNAMS, FRCP Professor, Department of Anaesthesiology, Teerthanker Mahaveer Medical College (TMMC), Moradabad, Uttar Pradesh, India

Dalim Kumar Baidya, MD Professor and HOD, Department of Anesthesiology, Critical Care and Pain Medicine, All India Institute of Medical Sciences (AIIMS), Guwahati, Assam, India

Pooja Bihani, MD, DNB, FIPA, PGDHM Associate Professor, Department of Anaesthesiology, All India Institute of Medical Sciences, Bhubaneswar, Odisha, India

Ghansham Biyani, MD, DNB, MNAMS, EDAIC Associate Professor, Department of Anesthesiology, All India Institute of Medical Sciences (AIIMS), Mangalagiri, Andhra Pradesh, India

Swati Chhabra, MD Additional Professor, Department of Anaesthesia and Critical Care, All India Institute of Medical Sciences (AIIMS), Jodhpur, Rajasthan, India

Nitin Choudhary, MD, DNB, MNAMS Assistant Professor, Department of Anaesthesiology, Pain Medicine and Critical Care, All India Institute of Medical Sciences (AIIMS), New Delhi, Delhi, India

Anita Chouhan, MD, PDFCA Assistant Professor, Department of Anesthesiology and Critical Care, All India Institute of Medical Sciences (AIIMS), Jodhpur, Rajasthan, India

Bhavna Gupta, DNB,MBA,FCCE,FNIV(Spain),FIMSA Associate Professor, Department of Anesthesiology, Critical Care and Pain, All India Institute of Medical Sciences, Rishikesh, Uttarakhand, India

Damarla Haritha, MD Assistant Professor, Department of Anesthesiology, Narayana Medical College, Nellore, Andhra Pradesh, India

Kamna Kakkar, MD, DNB, IDCCM, EDIAC Assistant Professor, Department of Anaesthesiology, Faculty of Medical and Health Sciences, SGT University, Gurugram, Haryana, India

Reshma Kalagara, MD Fellow PDCC Pain Medicine, All India Institute of Medical Sciences (AIIMS), Mangalagiri, Andhra Pradesh, India

Rakesh Kumar, MD Additional Professor, Department of Anaesthesia and Critical Care, All India Institute of Medical Sciences (AIIMS), Jodhpur, Rajasthan, India

Rohan Magoon, DM, MD Assistant Professor, Department of Anaesthesia, ABVIMS & Dr. RML Hospital, New Delhi, Delhi, India

Rajasekhar Metta, MD Assistant Professor, Department of Anaesthesia, All India Institute of Medical Sciences (AIIMS), Mangalagiri, Andhra Pradesh, India

Sadik Mohammed, MD, IDRA Additional Professor, Department of Anesthesiology and Critical Care, All India Institute of Medical Sciences (AIIMS), Jodhpur, Rajasthan, India

Naveen Paliwal, MD, PGDHM Professor, Department of Emergency Medicine, Dr. S.N. Medical College, Jodhpur, Rajasthan, India

Baby Pegu, MD Senior resident, Department of Anesthesiology, Critical Care and Pain Medicine, All India Institute of Medical Sciences (AIIMS), Guwahati, Assam, India

Soumya Sarkar, MD Assistant Professor, Department of Anesthesiology, All India Institute of Medical Sciences (AIIMS), Kalyani, West Bengal, India

Nageswara Rao Tangirala, Assistant Professor, Department of Anesthesiology, All India Institute of Medical Sciences (AIIMS), Mangalagiri, Andhra Pradesh, India

Kumari Tripta, MD Assistant Professor, Department of Anaesthesiology, Teerthanker Mahaveer Medical College (TMMC), Moradabad, Uttar Pradesh, India

Assessment of Acute Pain

1

Rajasekhar Metta and Reshma Kalagara

Abstract

Pain management is a crucial aspect of patient care in the perioperative period, as it can significantly impact a patient's recovery and overall well-being. The assessment of pain involves using various tools and techniques to evaluate the patient's pain experience. They are unidimensional pain scales, which primarily focus on pain intensity, and multidimensional pain scales, which consider various parameters to describe the pain characteristics. Multidimensional pain scales offer a more comprehensive understanding of the pain experience, encompassing sensory, affective, and functional aspects of pain, but may not be suitable for fast-paced environments. Effective communication with patients, along with the use of appropriate pain assessment tools, is essential for tailoring pain management strategies to individual needs, ultimately leading to improved patient satisfaction and outcomes.

R. Metta (✉)
Department of Anaesthesia, All India Institute of Medical Sciences (AIIMS), Mangalagiri, Andhra Pradesh, India

R. Kalagara
PDCC Pain Medicine, All India Institute of Medical Sciences (AIIMS), Mangalagiri, Andhra Pradesh, India

P. Ahluwalia (ed.), *Handbook of Perioperative Analgesia*,
https://doi.org/10.1007/978-981-96-7822-8_1

Keywords

Assessment of acute pain · Perioperative pain · Unidimensional scales · Multidimensional scales

Key Points

- Acute pain serves as a vital warning sign of injury or illness.
- Post-operative pain often limits the patient's functionality and recovery.
- Assessment of pain is of paramount importance in acute pain services. It is crucial for ensuring timely and effective pain management.
- Assessment of pain can be done using unidimensional, multidimensional, or behavioral assessment tools.
- It also reduces the risk of complications, such as chronic pain development, promotes faster recovery, and improves patient satisfaction.
- Regular pain evaluation fosters patient satisfaction by addressing their comfort and well-being during the acute phase.

1.1 Introduction

Margo McCaffery quoted that "Pain is whatever the experiencing person says it is, existing whenever he says it does" [1]. This phrase has laid the foundation of the idea of self-reporting of pain and formed the cornerstone of pain assessment. International Association for the Study of Pain (IASP) defined pain as "an unpleasant sensory and emotional experience associated with, or resembling that associated with, actual or potential tissue damage" [2]. This definition evolved the contemporary idea of pain as a complex and multifaceted experience which is significantly influenced by noxious, cognitive, and emotional factors.

Acute pain serves as a vital warning sign of injury or illness. Patients experience moderate to severe pain in the post-operative settings. Post-operative pain often limits the patient's functionality and recovery. Understanding and assessing acute pain is crucial in clinical practice, as it guides effective treatment strategies and improves patient outcomes. Anesthesiologists and pain physicians utilize a variety of tools and methods, such as self-report scales, observational methods, and physiological measures to evaluate pain characteristics, including its intensity, location, duration, and associated symptoms. This helps in the identification of the underlying causes of pain and facilitates the development of personalized pain management plans. This chapter aims to provide comprehensive insights and knowledge essential for effective evaluation of acute pain.

1.2 Types of Pain

A pain prescription can be made based on the expected intensity of pain after the procedure and the possible analgesic requirement. However, this isn't enough for effectively managing the pain. Identifying the type of pain during assessment is essential for effective pain management. Different types of pain require distinct treatment approaches. For example, nociceptive pain responds to NSAIDs or opioids, while neuropathic pain requires medications like gabapentinoids, anticonvulsants, or antidepressants. Accurate identification helps pinpoint the underlying cause of pain, guiding diagnosis and ensuring appropriate interventions. It also aids in tailoring treatment to the patient's specific needs, improving outcomes, minimizing complications, and enhancing patient satisfaction. Pain assessment without an attempt to understand the type of pain can lead to ineffective treatment, prolonged pain, or exacerbation of symptoms, making accurate assessment crucial for optimal care. Pain can be of the following types (Fig. 1.1) based on its origin, physical characteristics, and the mechanism behind it:

(a) *Nociceptive pain:* It is defined as an actual or threatened damage to the non-neural tissue activating the nociceptors. It can be somatic or visceral pain. Post-operative pain following laparotomies is often a combination of somatic and visceral pain [3]. The intensity of nociceptive pain usually comes down with time as the initial tissue insult resolves.

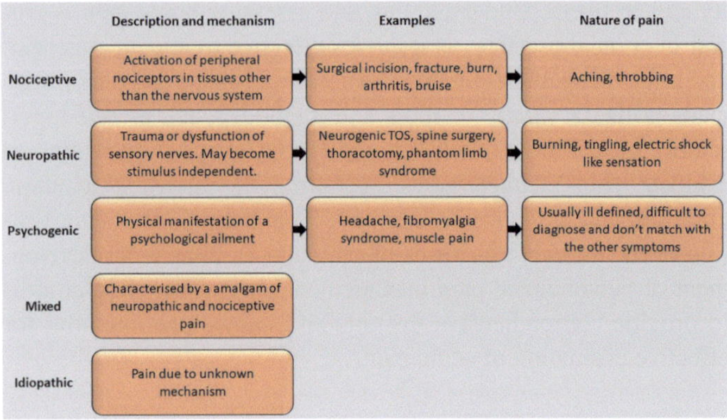

Fig. 1.1 Types of pain

(b) *Neuropathic pain:* It occurs secondary to injury of a sensory nerve. Injury to a nerve leads to peripheral and central sensitization which increases the risk of allodynia and hyperalgesia [4]. This makes the neuropathic pain to become stimulus independent in the later stages. Neuropathic pain can be seen post-operatively following thoracotomies, laparotomies, spine surgeries, surgeries on the brachial plexus [5].

(c) *Psychogenic pain:* It is a physical manifestation of a psychological ailment. Patients with depression and anxiety manifest psychogenic pain and are often associated with an increased risk of post-operative pain [6]. In these patients the intensity of pain will not match the underlying cause.

(d) *Mixed pain:* Mixed pain exhibits characteristics of different types of pain and originates from a myriad of mechanisms. The patients with mixed pain display the symptoms of both somatic pain and neuropathic pain.

(e) *Idiopathic pain:* It is a term given to describe pain where there is no identifiable physical or mental mechanism. A comprehensive evaluation should be performed to exclude the possible conditions before labelling pain as idiopathic.

1.3 Tools for Assessment

(a) *Unidimensional pain scales:* These scales are used for quick assessment of pain and focus on the intensity of pain as the single dimension of evaluation. Assessment using these scales is of limited use in complex pain scenarios [7]. A summary of the advantages and disadvantages of various unidimensional scales is provided in Table 1.1.

Table 1.1 Unidimensional pain scales

Scale	Advantages	Disadvantages
Numerical rating scale (NRS)	It can be presented visually or verbally It is highly sensitive to changes in pain intensity induced by treatment It is useful for differentiating pain intensity at rest and during activity It is valid and reliable in both younger and older patients	Lacks reliability in multi-dimensional aspects of complex pain scenarios Unreliable in patients like elderly, pediatric patients
Verbal descriptor scale (VDS)	Simple to describe	Must be presented in printed form Needs basic linguistic skills
Iowa pain thermometer (IPT)	Simple to describe Easy to use	Must be presented in printed form
Visual analogue scale (VAS)	The procedure is easy to understand and can be done quickly It can be repeated multiple times on the same patient	Lacks accuracy and sensitivity. Less reliable for immediate postoperative patients with cognitive impairment Description of assessment may confuse the patient
Faces pain scale (FPS)	Easy to use and understand Useful in patients with communication barriers	Difficult to determine whether pain or mood is being measured Must be presented in printed form

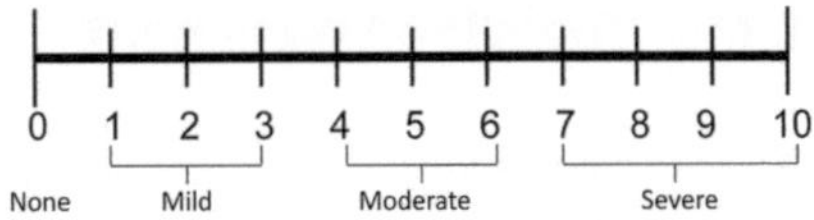

Fig. 1.2 Numeric rating scale

Numeric rating scale (NRS): NRS is a linear scale with 11 points ranging from 0–10. The two end points of the scale represents extremes of pain (Fig. 1.2). It can be represented to the patient either verbally or by using a simple visual aid. It is easy to understand and can be used in all patient above seven years age. It is sensitive tool to assess the change in intensity of pain following treatment. Presence of cognitive impairment and inability to communicate make it difficult for us to use this scale.

Verbal descriptor scale (VDS): VDS is composed of four to six adjectives which distinctively describe increasing levels pain intensity. The commonly used set of adjectives are no pain, mild pain, moderate pain, severe pain, very severe pain, worst possible pain, and no pain, mild pain, discomforting, distressing, horrible, excruciating pain [8]. The terms Verbal rating scale and Simple descriptive scale are often used interchangeably with VDS. The patient needs to have basic linguistic skills and the ability to identify the adjective best suited for the intensity of pain he is experiencing. So, the accuracy of this scale is not reliable (Fig. 1.3).

Iowa pain thermometer (IPT): IPT is an adjunct tool to VDS where in addition to the adjectives it has a diagram of a thermometer. The increasing temperature in this thermometer is analogous to the discomfort associated with the increasing intensity of pain (Fig. 1.4).

Visual analogue scale (VAS): It is widely used in research and clinical setting. It is composed of a straight line with one end marked as "no pain" and the other end marked as "worst possible pain" (Fig. 1.5). The patient should mark this line with a dot or mark with a finger on a point which corresponds to the present intensity of pain. Some VAS scales are made of slide rules with a movable line that can be placed at a point which

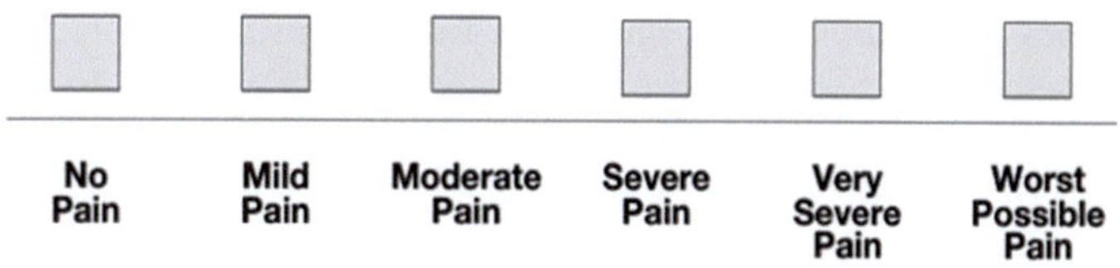

Fig. 1.3 Verbal descriptor scale

Fig. 1.4 Iowa pain thermometer

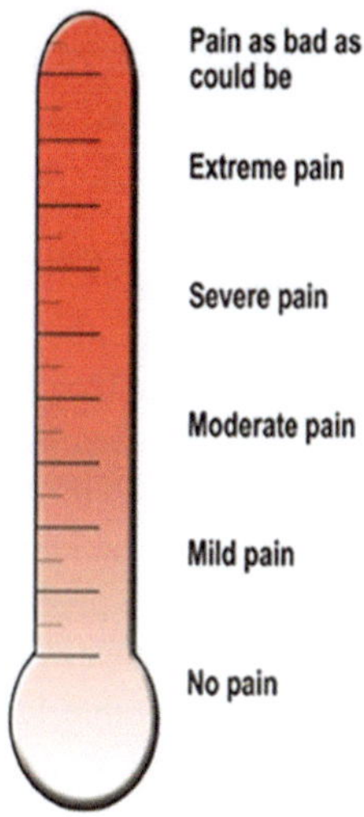

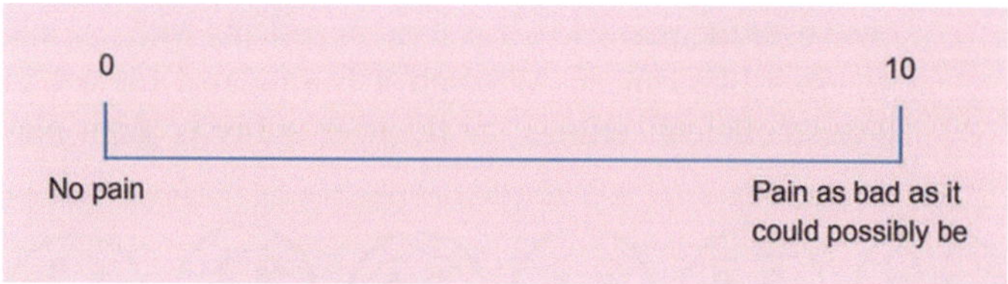

Fig. 1.5 Visual analogue scale

matches the pain intensity. It is ideal to mark these points to assess pain at rest and pain with movement. Lack of cues causes less confusion while using this scale. To improve the accuracy, patients can be instructed on how to use this scale for assessment of pain intensity preoperatively [9].

Faces pain scale (FPS): The Wong-Baker faces rating scale is widely used in pediatric settings across the globe. It has a series of six faces with a happy and smiling face at one end representing "no pain" and sad face with tears in the eyes at the other end representing severe pain (Fig. 1.6). Though this scale is originally described for use in pediatric population, there is recent evidence supporting its use in cognitively impaired and non-verbal adults [10]. There are several modified versions of FPS with variations in cheeks, lips, nose, and eyes to show the facial expressions associated with pain. In the revised faces pain scale (FPS-R), the childlike faces are replaced by faces of grown-up. In FPS-R, the face with no pain is represented by a neutral face instead of a happy smiling face and the teary-eyed face for severe pain is replaced by a frowning face (Fig. 1.7) [11].

(b) *Multidimensional pain scales:* These scales consider multiple parameters to describe the pain characteristics. Self-reports from the patients and the clinician's expertise are combined during the process of assessing the pain. The advantages and disadvantages of various multidimensional scales are summarized in Table 1.2.

Brief pain inventory (BPI): The tool consists of questions focusing on pain intensity and its interference with daily activities—designed to capture the patient's pain experience over the past 24 h. It is used in patients with chronic illnesses like cancer. Although it is validated for use in diverse clinical settings, its frequent utility is often hin-

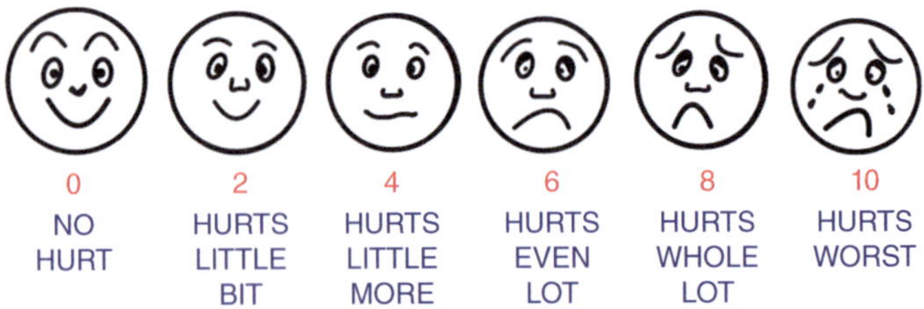
0
NO HURT
2
HURTS LITTLE BIT
4
HURTS LITTLE MORE
6
HURTS EVEN LOT
8
HURTS WHOLE LOT
10
HURTS WORST

Fig. 1.6 Wong-Baker faces pain rating scale

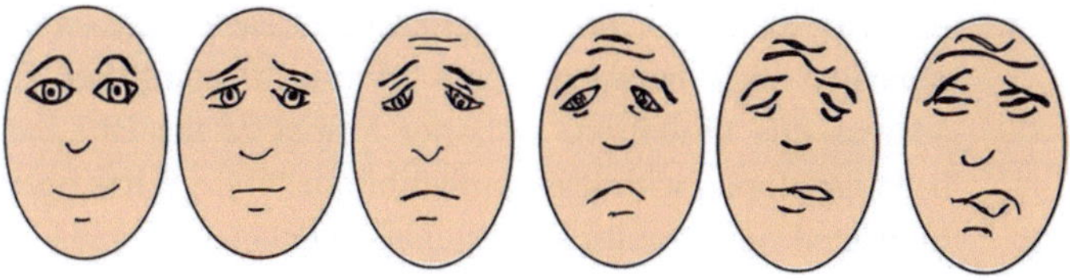

Fig. 1.7 Revised faces pain scales

Table 1.2 Multidimensional pain scales

Scale	Advantages	Disadvantages
Brief pain inventory (BPI)	Focused on pain intensity and pain's interference with function over 24 h period Validated in different groups of patients experiencing acute pain Available in multiple regional languages	It takes 5–15 min to complete making it less desirable for repeated use
Initial pain assessment tool (IPAT)	Tool can be used verbally or visually Can be completed by a physician or a nurse Includes diagram for site of pain Includes effects of pain on quality of life Useful for acute and chronic pain assessment Useful for detecting changes in pain symptoms following therapeutic intervention	Time consuming Does not consider emotional and psychological factors for pain in sufficient detail Not suitable for all patient populations
Mc gill pain questionnaire (MPQ)	Useful for assessment of acute and chronic pain Employs large varied word descriptors to assess sensory, affective, and evaluate dimensions of pain Measures both subjective quality and quantity of pain experience	Lengthy and complex Frequent assessments not possible Difficult to understand by patients High levels of anxiety and psychological disturbances can impair discriminative capacity

dered by caregiver non-compliance, as each assessment typically takes between 5 and 15 min to complete. To address this limitation, a shorter format of the BPI has been developed with less number of questions. It has been translated into multiple regional languages making it widely accessible.

Initial pain assessment tool (IPAT): IPAT captures a comprehensive range of pain-related information, including the pain's characteristics, the patient's expression of pain, aggravating and relieving factors, and the impact of pain on daily activities. It also provides a body diagram where patients can mark the locations of pain. The tool records the patient's acceptable pain level and utilizes a unidimensional pain scale for assessment to record the current pain intensity. IPAT is versatile and can be used to evaluate both acute and chronic pain, as well as to monitor changes in pain intensity following therapeutic interventions (Fig. 1.8).

The OLD CART acronym: It is an acronym for guiding a systematic approach for taking history of pain as a symptom. It stands for Onset, Location, Duration, Characteristics, Aggravating factors, Relieving factors, and Treatment. It should be used along with a unidimensional scale to know the intensity of pain.

Mc Gill Pain Questionnaire (MPQ): Developed by Dr. Ronald Melzack in 1975, MPQ is a comprehensive tool used to assess the sensory and emotional dimensions of pain. It consists of a series of sections, including a list of descriptive words for patients to characterize their pain (e.g., sharp, throbbing, burning); a pain intensity scale; and questions about the pain's duration, onset, and pattern. Additionally, the questionnaire includes a diagram where patients can mark the areas of pain on their body (Fig. 1.9). By capturing both the qualitative and quantitative aspects of pain, the MPQ provides a detailed understanding of a patient's pain experience, making it useful in clinical settings for diagnosis, treatment planning, and tracking changes in pain over time [12].

Fig. 1.8 Initial pain assessment tool

Initial Pain Assessment Tool

- PATIENT'S NAME ______ • DATE ______
- AGE / SEX ______ • ROOM ______
- DIAGNOSIS ______ • NURSE ______
- PHYSICIAN ______

① LOCATION : Patient or nurse marks drawing :

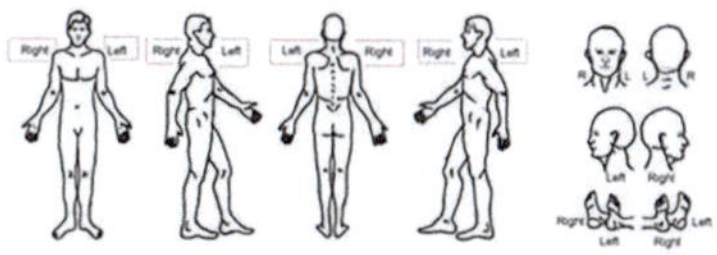

② INTENSITY : Patient rates the pain
Scale used : ______

Present pain ______ Worst pain gets ______
Best pain gets ______ Acceptable level of pain ______

③ Is This Pain Constant ? YES ______
No ______
If not, then how often does it occur ?

④ QUALITY : ______

⑤ ONSENT, DURATION, VARIATIONS, RHYTHMS : ______

⑥ MANNER OF EXPRESSING PAIN : ______

⑦ WHAT RELIEVES PAIN ? ______

⑧ WHAT CAUSES OR INCREASES THE PAIN ? ______

⑨ EFFECTS OF PAIN : ______

- Accompanying symptoms (eg. nausea)
- Sleep
- Appetite
- Physical Activity
- Relationship with others (eg. irritability)
- Emotions (eg. anger, suicidal, crying)
- Concentration
- Other

⑩ OTHER COMMENTS : ______

⑪ PLAN : ______

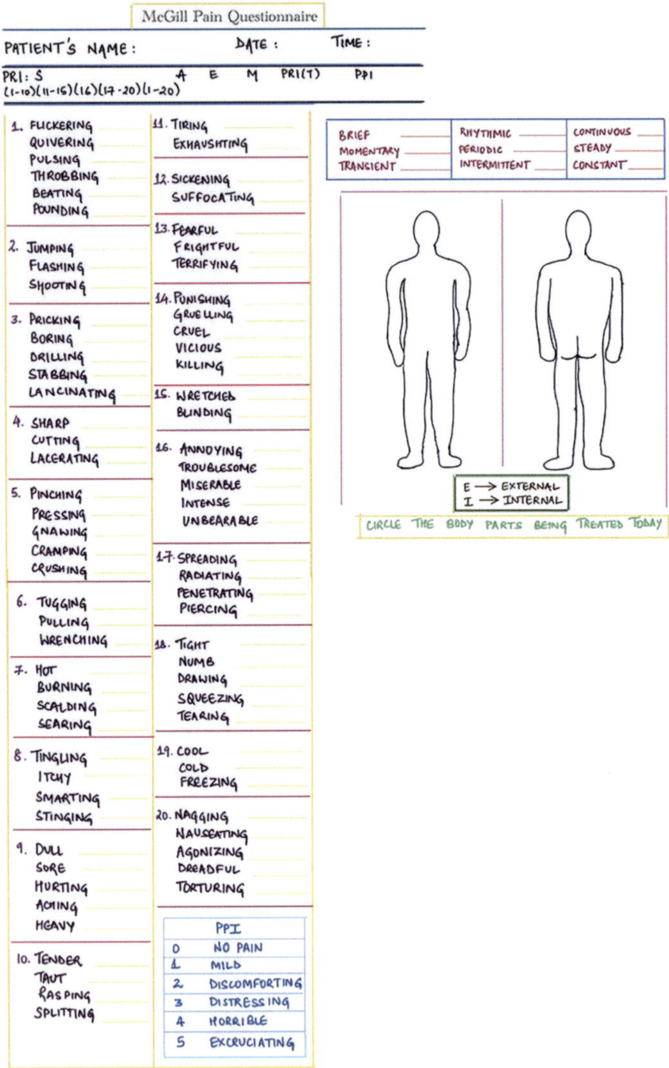

Fig. 1.9 Mc Gill Pain Questionnaire

(c) *Behavioral/observational pain assessment tools:* Behavioral observational pain assessment tools are designed to assess pain in individuals who are unable to communicate verbally, such as infants, young children, or patients with cognitive impairments. These tools rely on observing behavioral indicators—such as facial expressions, body movements, vocalizations, and physiological responses (e.g., heart rate, sweating)—to gauge the presence and intensity of pain.

Pain Assessment in Advanced Dementia Scale (PAINAD): The assessment of pain in advanced dementia is extremely challenging and complex, often resulting in under-treatment and poor pain management. The PAINAD scale is used to assess pain in individuals with advanced dementia. It evaluates five domains: breathing, negative vocalization, facial expression, body language, and consolability, with scores ranging from 0 to 2 for each (Fig. 1.10). The total score (0–10) reflects the intensity of pain, helping caregivers and healthcare providers identify and manage pain in non-verbal patients, improving their comfort and care [13].

FLACC scale: The FLACC scale (Face, Legs, Activity, Cry, Consolability) is a tool to evaluate pain in infants, young children, or individuals who cannot communicate verbally. It

Items*	0	1	2	Score
Breathing independent of vocalization	Normal	Occasional labored breathing. Short period of hyperventilation.	Noisy labored breathing. Long period of hyperventilation. Cheyne-Stokes respirations	
Negative vocalization	None	Occasional moan or groan. Low-level speech with a negative or disapproving quality.	Repeated troubled calling out. Loud moaning or groaning. Crying.	
Facial expression	Smiling or inexpressive	Sad. Frightened. Frown.	Facial grimacing.	
Body language	Relaxed	Tense. Distressed pacing. Fidgeting.	Rigid. Fists clenched. Knees pulled up. Pulling or pushing away. Striking out.	
Consolability	No need to console	Distracted or reassured by voice or touch.	Unable to console, distract or reassure.	
			Total**	

*Five-item observational tool (see the description of each item below).

**Total scores range from 0 to 10 (based on a scale of 0 to 2 for five items), with a higher score indicating more severe pain (0="no pain" to 10="severe pain").

Fig. 1.10 Pain Assessment In Advanced Dementia Scale (PAINAD)

assesses five categories: facial expression, leg movement, activity level, cry, and consolability, with each category scored from 0 to 2 (Fig. 1.11). The patient should be observed with body and legs uncovered for 2–3 min. An asleep child should be observed for at least 5 minutes. The total score ranges from 0 to 10, with higher scores indicating more intense pain. A total score of 1–3 indicates mild discomfort, 4–6 indicated moderate pain, and a score of above 7 indicates severe pain [14].

Critical Care Pain Observation Tool (CPOT): The CPOT is a pain assessment scale used to evaluate pain in critical care settings. It is designed for patients who cannot communicate due to sedation, intubation, or cognitive impairments. The CPOT assesses four key behavioral indicators: facial expression, body movements, muscle tension, and ventilator compliance (Fig. 1.12). Each category is scored from 0 to 2, with higher scores indicating more severe pain [15].

Doloplus-2 scale: The Doloplus-2 pain assessment scale is used to evaluate pain in elderly patients and individuals with cognitive impairments or dementia. The scale assesses pain through a combination of behavioral and physiological indicators, focusing on five key domains: somatic pain (physical signs),

Behaviour	0	1	2
Face	No particular expression or smile	Occasional grimace or frown, withdrawn, disinterested	Frequent to constant quivering chin, clenched jow
Legs	Normal position or relaxed	Uneasy, restless, tense	Kicking or legs drawn up
Activity	Lying quietly, normal position, moves easily	Squirming, shifting, back and forth, tense	Arched, rigid or jerking
Cry	No cry (awake or asleep)	Moans or whimpers; occasional complaint	Crying steadily, screams, sobs, frequent complaints
Consolability	Content, relaxed	Reassured by touching, hugging or being talked to, distractible	Difficul

Fig. 1.11 Face, Legs, Activity, Cry, Consolability (FLACC) scale

The Critical-Care Pain Observation Tool (CPOT)
(Adapted from Gélinas et al., AJCC 2006; 15(4):420-427)

Indicator	Score		Description
Facial expressions	Relaxed, neutral	0	No muscle tension observed
	Tense	1	Presence of frowning, brow lowering, orbit tightening and levator contraction or any other change (e.g. opening eyes or tearing during nociceptive procedures)
	Grimacing	2	All previous facial movements plus eyelid tightly closed (the patient may present with mouth open or biting the endotracheal tube)
Body movements	Absence of movements or normal position	0	Does not move at all (doesn't necessarily mean absence of pain) or normal position (movements not aimed toward the pain site or not made for the purpose of protection)
	Protection	1	Slow, cautious movements, touching or rubbing the pain site, seeking attention through movements
	Restlessness/Agitation	2	Pulling tube, attempting to sit up, moving limbs/thrashing, not following commands, striking at staff, trying to climb out of bed
Compliance with the ventilator (intubated patients)	Tolerating ventilator or movement	0	Alarms not activated, easy ventilation
	Coughing but tolerating	1	Coughing, alarms may be activated but stop spontaneously
	Fighting ventilator	2	Asynchrony: blocking ventilation, alarms frequently activated
OR **Vocalization (extubated patients)**	Talking in normal tone or no sound	0	Talking in normal tone or no sound
	Sighing, moaning	1	Sighing, moaning
	Crying out, sobbing	2	Crying out, sobbing
Muscle tension Evaluation by passive flexion and extension of upper limbs when patient is at rest or evaluation when patient is being turned	Relaxed	0	No resistance to passive movements
	Tense, rigid	1	Resistance to passive movements
	Very tense or rigid	2	Strong resistance to passive movements or incapacity to complete them
TOTAL		___/8	

Reproduced with permission.
For more information about the CPOT use, contact the author at celine.gelinas@mcgill.ca

*Note: when a patient's CPOT is > 3, the team will evaluate pain sources and modify/enhance pain management. CPOT sensitivity=86% and specificity=78% (Gelinas C, J Pain Sympt Man 2009).

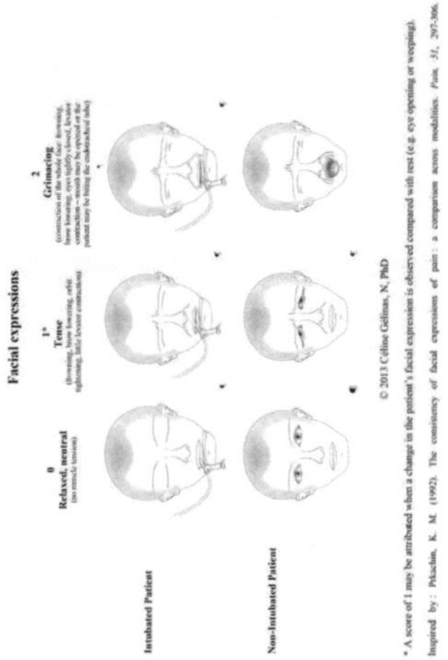

Fig. 1.12 Critical Care Pain Observation Tool (CPOT)

psychological pain (emotional responses), social pain (impact on social interactions), verbal pain expression (speech-related cues), and general discomfort (observable discomfort behaviors). Each domain is scored on a scale, and the total score provides a comprehensive assessment of the patient's pain intensity (Fig. 1.13). The Doloplus-2 is widely used in clinical settings to ensure that pain in vulnerable populations is accurately identified and managed, helping to improve their comfort and quality of life [16].

Checklist of Nonverbal Pain Indicators (CNPI): It evaluates behaviors and physical signs, including facial expression, vocalizations, body movements, changes in interactions, and physiological signs like vital changes. The CNPI helps healthcare providers identify pain in nonverbal patients, enabling timely and appropriate pain management (Fig. 1.14) [17].

DOLOPLUS-2 SCALE

BEHAVIOURAL PAIN ASSESSMENT IN THE ELDERLY

NAME : Christian name :

Unit :

Behavioural records

Behavioural records		DATES			
SOMATIC REACTIONS					
1• Somatic complaints	• no complaint	0	0	0	0
	• complaints expressed upon inquiry only	1	1	1	1
	• occasional involuntary complaints	2	2	2	2
	• continuous involuntary complaints	3	3	3	3
2• Protective body postures adopted at rest	• no protective body posture	0	0	0	0
	• the patient occasionally avoids certain postures	1	1	1	1
	• protective postures continuously and effectively sought	2	2	2	2
	• protective postures continuously sought, without success	3	3	3	3
3• Protection of sore areas	• no protective action taken	0	0	0	0
	• protective actions attempted without interfering against any investigation or nursing	1	1	1	1
	• protective actions against any investigations and nursing	2	2	2	2
	• protective actions taken at rest, even when not approached	3	3	3	3
4• Expression	• usual expression	0	0	0	0
	• expression showing pain when approached	1	1	1	1
	• expression showing pain even without being approached	2	2	2	2
	• permanent and unusually blank look (voiceless, staring, looking blank)	3	3	3	3
5• Sleep pattern	• normal sleep	0	0	0	0
	• difficult to go to sleep	1	1	1	1
	• frequent waking (restlessness)	2	2	2	2
	• insomnia affecting waking times	3	3	3	3
PSYCHOMOTOR REACTIONS					
6• Activities of daily living (washing &/or dressing)	• usual abilities unaffected	0	0	0	0
	• usual abilities slightly affected (careful but thorough)	1	1	1	1
	• usual abilities highly impaired, washing &/or dressing is laborious and incomplete	2	2	2	2
	• washing &/or dressing rendered impossible as the patient resists any attempt	3	3	3	3
7• Mobility	• usual abilities & activities remain unaffected	0	0	0	0
	• usual activities are reduced (the patient avoids certain movements and reduces his/her walking distance)	1	1	1	1
	• usual activities and abilities reduced (even with help, the patient cuts down on his/her movements)	2	2	2	2
	• any movement is impossible, the patient resists all persuasion	3	3	3	3
PSYCHOSOCIAL REACTIONS					
8• Communication	• unchanged	0	0	0	0
	• heightened (the patient demands attention in an unusual manner)	1	1	1	1
	• lessened (the patient cuts him/herself off)	2	2	2	2
	• absence or refusal of any form of communication	3	3	3	3
9• Social life	• participates normally in every activity (meals, entertainment, therapy workshops)	0	0	0	0
	• participates in activities when asked to do so only	1	1	1	1
	• sometimes refuses to participate in any activity	2	2	2	2
	• refuses to participate in anything	3	3	3	3
10• Problems of behaviour	• normal behaviour	0	0	0	0
	• problems of repetitive reactive behaviour	1	1	1	1
	• problems of permanent reactive behaviour	2	2	2	2
	• permanent behaviour problems (without any external stimulus)	3	3	3	3
	SCORE				

Fig. 1.13 Doloplus-2

For: Adults who are nonverbal; designed to measure pain behaviors in cognitively impaired older adults.

Scoring: Score each item both on movement and at rest. Score "0" if the behavior was not observed. Score "1" if the behavior occurred even briefly. Subtotal the scores for the movement column and the at rest column. Add them together for a total score. There are no clear cut-off scores to indicate severity of pain. Instead, the presence of any of these behaviors may be indicative of pain and warrants further investigation, treatment and/or monitoring.

CHECKLIST OF NONVERBAL PAIN INDICATORS (CNPI)		
Behavior	**Movement**	**At Rest**
1. Vocal complaints: nonverbal Sighs, gasps, moans, groans, cries		
2. Facial grimaces/winces Furrowed brow, narrowed eyes, clenched teeth, tightened lips, jaw drop, distorted expressions		
3. Bracing Clutching or holding onto furniture, equipment or affected area during movement		
4. Restlessness Constant or intermittent shifting of position, rocking, intermittent or constant hand motions, inability to keep still		
5. Rubbing Massaging affected area		
6. Vocal complaints: verbal Words expressing discomfort or pain, e.g. "ouch," "that hurts"; cursing during movement; exclamations of protest, e.g. "stop," "that's enough"		
Subtotal Scores		
Total Score		

Feldt KS. The checklist of nonverbal pain indicators (CNPI). Pain Manag Nurs. 2000 Mar.1(1):13-21.

Fig. 1.14 Checklist of Nonverbal Pain Indicators (CNPI)

Pain Assessment for the Dementing Elderly (PADE) scale: This scale considers several non-verbal observable behaviors and physiological signs of pain, such as facial expressions, body movements, vocalizations, and changes in interactions with others. The PADE scale includes categories like facial grimacing, body tension, and irritability, with scores that help clinicians gauge the intensity of pain (Fig. 1.15) [18].

Tool	Pain Assessment for the Dementing Elderly (PADE)
Tool developers	Villanueva, M.R., Smith, T.L., Erickson, J.S., Lee, A.C., Singer, C.M.
Purpose	The Pain Assessment for the Dementing Elderly (PADE) is an informant-based tool for the assessment of pain in individuals with advanced dementia. It was developed to help caregivers assess patient behaviour that may indicate pain.
Conceptual basis	The terms distress and pain are used interchangeably. Association between pain and agitation was noted. Pain assessment by observation rests upon three key assumptions: 1. Facial characteristics, body posture and movement patterns can indicate the presence of pain. 2. Pain can interfere with activities of daily living (ADLs) such as dressing and eating. 3. Caregivers can reliably observe and rate behaviour. Assumptions reflect a conceptual basis for pain by observation of behaviours.
Item Generation	Item generation is based on - literature review (Kovach: facial features and ADL) - interviews with nursing staff at care facilities - naturalistic observation by research associates (logged 30 hours over a 2-week period in a dementia care unit). Tool items 24 items in three parts: I Physical - observable facial expression - breathing pattern - posture II Global Assessment- proxy evaluation of pain intensity III Functional (ADL) - dressing - feeding oneself - transfers from wheelchair to bed. Items were validated by clinical experts in three settings. Feedback was provided by staff regarding ease of use, comprehensiveness and manual instructions. Adjustments were made.
Content Validity	The PADE has not been subjected to content validation by independent experts in pain in elders with dementia. However, subsequent studies have indicated that the tool is sensitive to pain behaviours

Fig. 1.15 Pain Assessment for the Dementing Elderly (PADE) scale

1.4 Review of Literature

(a) Multidimensional and unidimensional scales
This systematic review by Crisman E et al. [19], compared multidimensional and unidimensional pain scales in the acute care setting to assess patients' analgesic needs. Few studies that directly compared the two scale types suggested that multidimensional scales are better in capturing the complexity of pain and patient preferences, potentially reducing opioid use. However, it has been observed that the use of multidimensional scales in the ED is limited due to the longer time it may take for the assessment. This highlights the practical difficulty one faces with these tools in fast-paced environments. Moreover, the available data comparing multidimensional and unidimensional scales is limited. Further research should aim to develop accurate tools which consider pain as a multifaceted entity and aid in faster assessment in perioperative settings. In a systematic review by Baamer RM et al. [7], no evidence is found suggesting that one unidimensional scale is superior to other in assessing postoperative pain.

(b) Assessment in elderly
Kim YS and colleagues [20] studied the tools for assessing pain in elderly patients irrespective of the presence of cognitive impairment. They reviewed 41 publications in which they found that self-reporting pain is considered the gold standard, and the NRS, VAS, FPS, and VDS being valid methods for the elderly with no cognitive dysfunction. For those with dementia, behavioral observations provide a valuable alternative for pain assessment. Facial expressions, verbalizations/vocalizations, body language, changes in activity patterns, alterations in mental status, and variations in interpersonal interactions are identified to be the key pain behaviors. Validated tools for observational pain assessment in acute care include Doloplus-2, PAINAD, PADE, and CNPI scales. But these scales typically require around 1–12 min for completion. Elderly patients have access to treatment in diverse

environments such as hospitals, long-term care facilities, clinics, and even their own homes. Pain evaluation in these settings may also involve caregivers or family members, not just healthcare professionals. Therefore, pain assessment should extend beyond medical staff alone. To ensure effective and timely medical intervention, there is a clear need for a reliable, quick-to-implement pain assessment tool tailored for older adults that works across different settings and is not reliant on specific caregivers.

(c) Adjunctive tools for neuropathic pain
Neuropathic pain remains a significant therapeutic challenge for pain specialists. In a study by Jensen MP et al. [21], the Neuropathic Pain Scales (NPS) were used to assess the complexities of neuropathic pain in 159 patients with diabetic foot. The study found that the NPS is effective in characterizing the multidimensional nature of neuropathic pain and in tracking changes in pain characteristics with treatment. Similarly, Bennett MI et al. [22] investigated the utility of the Self-Report Leeds Assessment of Neuropathic Symptoms and Signs (S-LANSS) scale (Fig. 1.16) for identifying neuropathic pain. They found that the S-LANSS scale correctly identified 75% of pain types when self-completed and 80% when administered in an interview format. While there is substantial evidence supporting the use of various scales for identifying neuropathic pain, their application in the perioperative setting remains limited, highlighting the need for further research in this area.

(d) Impact on multimodal analgesia and opioid usage
Pain assessment plays a vital role in healthcare, particularly in surgical and postoperative care, by guiding the pain management strategies and improving patient outcomes. Accurate assessment allows clinicians to personalize pain treatment, optimizing the use of multimodal analgesia (MMA) to reduce reliance on opioids while ensuring effective pain relief [23]. This approach not only minimizes opioid-related risks, such as nausea and respiratory depression, but also supports faster recovery and fewer complications. Regular pain assessments enable real-time adjustments to

1.	**In the area where you have pain, do you also have "pins and needles", tingling or prickling sensations?**	
	☐ NO – I don't get these sensations	0
	☐ YES – I get these sensations	5
2.	**Does the painful area change colour (perhaps look mottled or more red) when the pain is particularly bad?**	
	☐ NO – The pain does not affect the colour of my skin	0
	☐ YES – I have noticed that the pain does make my skin look different from normal.	5
3.	**Does your pain make the affected skin abnormally sensitive to touch? Getting unpleasant sensations or pain when lightly stroking the skin might describe this.**	
	☐ NO – The pain does not make my skin abnormally sensitive to touch.	0
	☐ YES – My skin in that area is particularly sensitive to touch.	3
4.	**Does your pain come on suddenly and in bursts for no apparent reason when you are completely still? Words like "electric shocks", jumping and bursting might describe this.**	
	☐ NO – My pain doesn't really feel like this.	0
	☐ YES – I get these sensations often.	2
5.	**In the area where you have pain, does your skin feel unusually hot like a burning pain?**	
	☐ NO – I don't have burning pain	0
	☐ YES – I get burning pain often	1
6.	**Gently rub the painful area with your index finger and then rub a non-painful area (for example, an area of skin further away or on the opposite side from the painful area). How does this rubbing feel in the painful area?**	
	☐ The painful area feels no different from the non-painful area	0
	☐ I feel discomfort, like pins and needles, tingling or burning in the painful area that is different from the non-painful area.	5
7.	**Gently press on the painful area with your finger tip and then gently press in the same way onto a non-painful area (the same non-painful area that you chose in the last question). How does this feel in the painful area?**	
	☐ The painful area does not feel different from the non-painful area.	0
	☐ I feel numbness or tenderness in the painful area that is different from the non-painful area.	3
	Total score:	

Fig. 1.16 Self-Report Leeds Assessment of Neuropathic Symptoms and Signs (S-LANSS) scale

treatment plans, preventing pain escalation and reducing the likelihood of opioid misuse. Beyond pain relief, proper assessment enhances patient satisfaction, accelerates recovery, and reduces hospital readmissions. Ultimately, effective pain management contributes to better clinical efficiency and long-term health outcomes [23].

(e) Impact on patient outcomes

Effective pain assessment and management are critical to enhancing postoperative recovery and preventing long-term complications. Adequate pain control facilitates early mobilization and physical therapy, essential components of Enhanced Recovery After Surgery (ERAS) protocols, which help reduce the risk of complications like deep vein thrombosis (DVT), pulmonary embolism (PE), and pneumonia [24, 25]. It also promotes better sleep, which is vital for healing, immune function, and overall recovery [26]. Timely and effective pain management in the early postoperative period is key to preventing central sensitization, a process where the nervous system becomes hypersensitive to pain, which can lead to chronic pain and disability [24]. Uncontrolled pain can also contribute to psychological distress, including anxiety, depression, and postoperative delirium, all of which can hinder recovery. By reducing these emotional burdens, effective pain management improves patient satisfaction and overall well-being. Furthermore, patients who experience optimal pain relief tend to have fewer complications, faster mobilization, and shorter hospital stays, leading to reduced healthcare costs. Well-managed pain not only enhances functional recovery but also lowers the risk of long-term disability, chronic pain syndromes, and readmissions, ultimately improving both short-term and long-term patient outcomes [24–28].

(f) Impact on Enhanced Recovery After Surgery (ERAS)

The Enhanced Recovery After Surgery (ERAS) protocol is an evidence-based approach designed to improve postoperative recovery, reduce complications, and enhance patient outcomes. Central to the success of ERAS is effective pain management, which minimizes opioid use, promotes early mobilization, and accelerates recovery. Pain assessment plays a vital role in personalizing pain management, guiding the use of multimodal analgesia (including regional anesthesia, non-opioid analgesics, and adjuvant medications) to reduce opioid consumption and its associated side effects [29]. Proper pain control also helps attenuate the stress response to surgery, speeding up recovery and reducing the risk of complications such as deep vein thrombosis and pulmonary embolism. By optimizing pain relief, ERAS protocols contribute to shorter hospital stays, fewer readmissions, and lower healthcare costs, while also improving patient satisfaction. Moreover, the use of multimodal analgesia reduces opioid use, lowering the risk of opioid-related complications and dependence, ultimately improving long-term outcomes [30].

(g) Impact on patient satisfaction
Effective pain management is closely linked to patient satisfaction, particularly in the postoperative setting where pain relief is often a primary concern. Studies consistently show that adequate pain control leads to higher satisfaction, as patients' expectations regarding pain relief significantly influence their perception of care. Inadequate pain management can result in frustration, negative feedback, and even legal action, highlighting the importance of timely and accurate pain assessments [31]. Effective communication plays a key role in managing expectations, with informed patients feeling more empowered and satisfied with their care. A patient-centered approach, which tailors pain management to individual preferences and values, further enhances satisfaction by giving patients a sense of control over their treatment [32]. Regular reassessments of pain ensure that treatment plans are continuously adjusted to meet the patient's evolving needs, contributing to a positive patient experience and improved outcomes [33].

(h) Impact on clinical efficiency
Pain assessment is crucial for improving clinical efficiency by enabling timely interventions, optimizing resource allocation, and reducing unnecessary treatments. Regular pain reassessment using scales like the Numerical Rating Scale (NRS) or Visual Analog Scale (VAS) allows healthcare providers to quickly identify inadequately controlled pain and adjust treatment plans accordingly, preventing delays in care and minimizing disruptions in clinical workflows [34]. This proactive approach leads to better patient outcomes, fewer complications, and more efficient use of hospital resources, ultimately

saving costs. Accurate pain management prevents unnecessary diagnostic tests and treatments by addressing pain early, avoiding the need for additional interventions [35]. Furthermore, effective pain control supports faster recovery, reduces hospital stays, and enhances hospital throughput, enabling healthcare systems to treat more patients efficiently and reduce readmissions, which further cuts costs [36].

(i) Impact on Chronic Post-Surgical Pain (CPSP)
Uncontrolled acute pain after surgery significantly increases the risk of developing CPSP, a complex condition influenced by factors such as pre-existing pain, poor acute pain management, and surgical technique. Inadequate perioperative pain control, particularly in the immediate postoperative phase, can lead to central sensitization, where the nervous system becomes hypersensitive to pain, potentially resulting in chronic pain. Pain assessment plays a crucial role in preventing CPSP by identifying high-risk patients and ensuring timely, effective pain management [37]. Early interventions like preemptive analgesia, regional nerve blocks, and gabapentinoids can help reduce the acute pain response and prevent its progression to chronic pain. Regular preoperative and postoperative pain assessments allow for tailored pain management strategies, improving long-term outcomes and reducing the risk of chronic pain development.

(j) Transitional Pain Services (TPS)
The TPS are designed to manage postoperative pain from the early recovery phase through to post-discharge, with a focus on preventing chronic pain and minimizing opioid use. Pain assessment is a central component of TPS, enabling personalized, dynamic pain management throughout recovery [38]. It helps identify high-risk patients, such as those with pre-existing chronic pain or substance use disorders, allowing for proactive, tailored pain management strategies. Regular assessments guide multimodal analgesia, helping adjust pain relief methods as needed and reducing reliance on opioids by facilitating opioid-sparing strategies. Figure 1.17 emphasizes the components of assessing pain. Pain assessment also plays a key role in preventing chronic pain by ensuring that acute

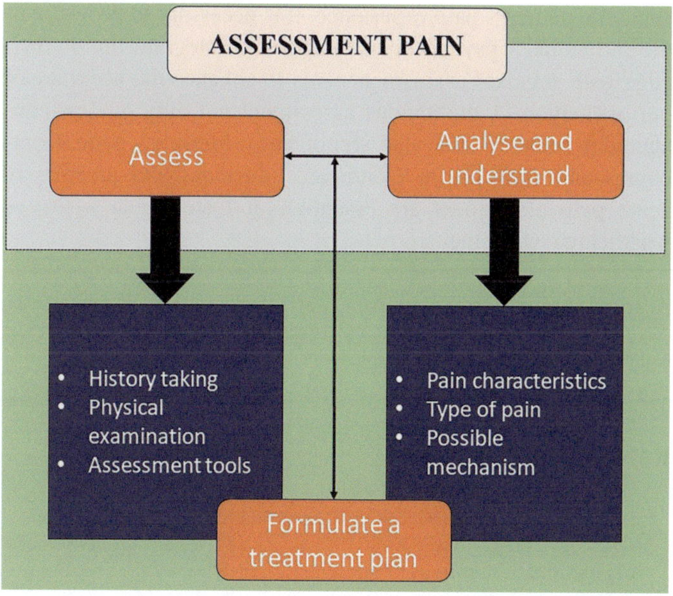

Fig. 1.17 Components of assessment of pain

pain is effectively managed early, reducing the risk of long-term pain and disability. Additionally, it supports opioid stewardship by guiding the tapering of opioids and identifying alternative pain management approaches. TPS includes follow-up care to monitor pain progression, address complications, and adjust treatment plans as necessary. Psychosocial factors, such as anxiety or depression, are also assessed, providing a holistic approach to pain management that reduces the risk of chronic pain development.

1.5 Conclusion

The assessment of acute pain is a critical component of effective patient care that requires a multifaceted approach. Anesthesiologists can utilize patient self-reports, comprehensive history-taking, and thorough physical examinations to understand the patient's pain experience. It is necessary to be aware of the individual's psychosocial factors and integrate this knowledge with standard assessment tools to enhance the accuracy of our evaluation. A meticulous assessment not only guides management strategies but also significantly improves patient outcomes and satisfaction. Continued education and practice in acute pain assessment are essential for fostering an effective healthcare environment.

Acknowledgement Dr. Vidya Tharu K MD, Fellowship in GI Anaesthesia, Assistant Professor, Department of Anaesthesiology, Seth G.S. Medical College and K.E.M. Hospital, Parel, Mumbai.

References

1. Remembering Margo McCaffery's contributions to pain management | Oncology Nursing Society. (2018, January 18). ONS. https://www.ons.org/publicationsresearch/voice/news-views/remembering-margo-mccafferys-contributions-pain-management#:~:text=McCaffery's%201968%20definition%20of%20pain,and%20treating%20patients%20in%20pain
2. Raja SN, Carr DB, Cohen M, Finnerup NB, Flor H, Gibson S, Keefe FJ, Mogil JS, Ringkamp M, Sluka KA, Song XJ, Stevens B, Sullivan MD, Tutelman PR, Ushida T, Vader K. The revised International Association for the Study of Pain definition of pain: concepts, challenges, and compromises. Pain. 2020;161(9):1976–82. https://doi.org/10.1097/j.pain.0000000000001939. PMID: 32694387; PMCID: PMC7680716.
3. Blichfeldt-Eckhardt MR, Ørding H, Andersen C, Licht PB, Toft P. Early visceral pain predicts chronic pain after laparoscopic cholecystectomy. PAIN®. 2014;155(11):2400–7.
4. Bhatia P, Metta R. Rebound pain: undesired, yet unexplored. J Anaesthesiol Clin Pharmacol. 2022;38(4):527–8.
5. Borsook D, Kussman BD, George E, Becerra LR, Burke DW. Surgically induced neuropathic pain: understanding the perioperative process. Ann Surg. 2013;257(3):403–12.
6. Gravani S, Matiatou M, Nikolaidis PT, Menenakos E, Zografos CG, Zografos G, Albanopoulos K. Anxiety and depression affect early postoperative pain dimensions after bariatric surgery. J Clin Med. 2020;10(1):53.
7. Baamer RM, Iqbal A, Lobo DN, Knaggs RD, Levy NA, Toh LS. Utility of unidimensional and functional pain assessment tools in adult postoperative patients: a systematic review. Br J Anaesth. 2022;128(5):874–88.

8. Gracely RH, Dubner R. Reliability and validity of verbal descriptor scales of painfulness. Pain. 1987;29(2):175–85.
9. Myles PS, Urquhart N. The linearity of the visual analogue scale in patients with severe acute pain. Anaesth Intensive Care. 2005;33(1):54–8.
10. Garra G, Singer AJ, Taira BR, Chohan J, Cardoz H, Chisena E, Thode HC Jr. Validation of the Wong-Baker FACES pain rating scale in pediatric emergency department patients. Acad Emerg Med. 2010;17(1):50–4.
11. Adeboye A, Hart R, Senapathi SH, Ali N, Holman L, Thomas HW. Assessment of functional pain score by comparing to traditional pain scores. Cureus. 2021;13(8)
12. Ngamkham S, Vincent C, Finnegan L, Holden JE, Wang ZJ, Wilkie DJ. The McGill pain questionnaire as a multidimensional measure in people with cancer: an integrative review. Pain Manag Nurs. 2012;13(1):27–51.
13. Felton N, Lewis JS, Cockburn SJ, Hodgson M, Dawson S. Pain assessment for individuals with advanced dementia in care homes: a systematic review. Geriatrics (Basel). 2021;6(4):101. https://doi.org/10.3390/geriatrics6040101. PMID: 34698157; PMCID: PMC8544573.
14. Voepel-Lewis T, Shayevitz JR, Malviya S. The FLACC: a behavioral scale for scoring postoperative pain in young children. Pediatr Nurs. 1997;23(3):293–7.
15. Nazari R, Froelicher ES, Nia HS, Hajihosseini F, Mousazadeh N. Diagnostic values of the critical care pain observation tool and the behavioral pain scale for pain assessment among unconscious patients: a comparative study. Ind J Crit Care Med. 2022;26(4):472.
16. Rostad HM, Utne I, Grov EK, Puts M, Halvorsrud L. Measurement properties, feasibility and clinical utility of the Doloplus-2 pain scale in older adults with cognitive impairment: a systematic review. BMC Geriatr. 2017;17:1–28.
17. Feldt KS. The checklist of nonverbal pain indicators (CNPI). Pain Manag Nurs. 2000;1(1):13–21.
18. Villanueva MR, Smith TL, Erickson JS, Lee AC, Singer CM. Pain assessment for the dementing elderly (PADE): reliability and validity of a new measure. J Am Med Dir Assoc. 2003;4(1):1–8.
19. Crisman E, Appenzeller-Herzog C, Tabakovic S, Nickel CH, Minotti B. Multidimensional versus unidimensional pain scales for the assessment of analgesic requirement in the emergency department: a systematic review. Intern Emerg Med. 2024;19:1–9.
20. Kim YS, Park JM, Moon YS, Han SH. Assessment of pain in the elderly: a literature review. Natl Med J India. 2017;30(4):203–7. https://doi.org/10.4103/0970-258X.218673. PMID: 29162753.
21. Jensen MP, Friedman M, Bonzo D, Richards P. The validity of the neuropathic pain scale for assessing diabetic neuropathic pain in a clinical trial. Clin J Pain. 2006;22(1):97–103.

22. Bennett MI, Smith BH, Torrance N, Potter J. The S-LANSS score for identifying pain of predominantly neuropathic origin: validation for use in clinical and postal research. J Pain. 2005;6(3):149–58.
23. Chou R, Gordon DB, de Leon-Casasola OA, et al. Management of postoperative pain: a clinical practice guideline from the American pain society, the American Society of Regional Anesthesia and Pain Medicine, and the American Society of Anesthesiologists' committee on regional anesthesia, executive committee, and administrative council. J Pain. 2016;17(2):131–57.
24. Kehlet H, Wilmore DW. Multimodal strategies to improve surgical outcome. Am J Surg. 2002;183(6):630–41.
25. Frassanito L, Vergari A, Nestorini R, Cerulli G, Placella G, Pace V, Rossi M. Enhanced recovery after surgery (ERAS) in hip and knee replacement surgery: description of a multidisciplinary program to improve management of the patients undergoing major orthopedic surgery. Musculoskelet Surg. 2020;104:87–92.
26. Rampes S, Ma K, Divecha YA, Alam A, Ma D. Postoperative sleep disorders and their potential impacts on surgical outcomes. J Biomed Res. 2020;34(4):271.
27. Woolf CJ. Neuropathic pain: a maladaptive response of the nervous system to damage. Annu Rev Neurosci. 2009;32:1–32.
28. Ferreira MS, Pereira MG. The mediator role of psychological morbidity in patients with chronic low back pain in differentiated treatments. J Health Psychol. 2014;19(9):1197–207.
29. Kaye AD, Urman RD, Rappaport Y, Siddaiah H, Cornett EM, Belani K, Salinas OJ, Fox CJ. Multimodal analgesia as an essential part of enhanced recovery protocols in the ambulatory settings. J Anaesthesiol Clin Pharmacol. 2019;35(Suppl 1):S40–5.
30. Ljungqvist O, Scott M, Fearon KC. Enhanced recovery after surgery: a review. JAMA Surg. 2017;152(3):292–8.
31. Subramanian P, Ramasamy S, Ng KH, Chinna K, Rosli R. Pain experience and satisfaction with postoperative pain control among surgical patients. Int J Nurs Pract. 2016;22(3):232–8.
32. Haverfield MC, Giannitrapani K, Timko C, Lorenz K. Patient-centered pain management communication from the patient perspective. J Gen Intern Med. 2018;33:1374–80.
33. Niemi-Murola L, Pöyhiä R, Onkinen K, Rhen B, Mäkelä A, Niemi TT. Patient satisfaction with postoperative pain management—effect of preoperative factors. Pain Manag Nurs. 2007;8(3):122–9.
34. Rose L, Smith O, Gélinas C, Haslam L, Dale C, Luk E, Burry L, McGillion M, Mehta S, Watt-Watson J. Critical care nurses' pain assessment and management practices: a survey in Canada. Am J Crit Care. 2012;21(4):251–9.
35. Rajan J, Behrends M. Acute pain in older adults: recommendations for assessment and treatment. Anesthesiol Clin. 2019;37(3):507–20.

36. Elvir-Lazo OL, White PF. The role of multimodal analgesia in pain management after ambulatory surgery. Curr Opin Anesthesiol. 2010;23(6):697–703.
37. Rosenberger DC, Pogatzki-Zahn EM. Chronic post-surgical pain–update on incidence, risk factors and preventive treatment options. BJA Educ. 2022;22(5):190–6.
38. Klimke R, Ott A, Romero CS, Berendes A, Urman RD, Luedi MM, Ashok V. Transitional pain service: an update. Curr Pain Headache Rep. 2024;28(6):457–64.

Pain Pathways: From Periphery to Perception

2

Swati Chhabra and Rakesh Kumar

Abstract

Pain is a complex sensory and emotional experience involving multiple pathways from peripheral detection to central perception. This chapter explores the pain pathway, starting from nociceptors in the periphery that detect mechanical, thermal, and chemical stimuli, progressing through transduction and transmission phases in the spinal cord, and culminating in perception within the brain. Neurotransmitters like glutamate and Substance P facilitate pain transmission, while inhibitory agents like GABA, norepinephrine, and endogenous opioids modulate and suppress these signals. The chapter also discusses critical elements in acute and chronic pain management, focusing on the modulation of neurotransmitter pathways to counteract pain sensitization. Additionally, classifications of pain types and mechanisms of peripheral and central sensitization are covered, highlighting recent therapeutic advancements aimed at targeting specific neurotransmitter pathways. This comprehensive view provides insights into potential treatment strategies for managing both acute and chronic pain conditions.

S. Chhabra (✉) · R. Kumar
Department of Anaesthesia and Critical Care, All India Institute of Medical Sciences (AIIMS), Jodhpur, Rajasthan, India

P. Ahluwalia (ed.), *Handbook of Perioperative Analgesia*,
https://doi.org/10.1007/978-981-96-7822-8_2

Keywords

Pain · Nociceptors · Neurotransmitters · Pain Perception · Pain Pathways · Sensitization

Key Points

- Pain perception aims to alert the body's defense system to respond to a stimulus to prevent additional tissue damage.
- Pain involves a complex interplay of physiological and psychological processes, spanning from the peripheral sensory receptors that detect harmful stimuli to the brain, where these stimuli are interpreted as pain.
- The primary purpose of the PNS, which is made up of nerves and ganglia outside the brain and spinal cord, is to link the CNS to our body's limbs and organs.
- In pain pathways, excitatory neurotransmitters like glutamate and Substance P transmit the initial pain signal, while inhibitory neurotransmitters like GABA, norepinephrine, and endogenous opioids work to suppress it.
- Disruptions in this balance are central to chronic pain and hyperalgesia. This complex interplay makes neurotransmitters a primary focus for pain management strategies and pharmacological interventions aimed at modulating the pain pathway.
- The process by which a noxious stimulus is perceived as pain by an individual happens in four steps, viz., transduction, transmission, modulation, and perception.

2.1 Introduction

Pain is one of the most fundamental sensations we experience, serving as a protective mechanism that alerts us to potential harm. Pain involves a complex interplay of physiological and psychological processes, spanning from the peripheral sensory receptors that detect harmful stimuli to the brain, where these stimuli are interpreted as pain. Understanding this pathway—commonly called the "pain pathway"—is crucial for deciphering how the body detects, transmits, and perceives pain.

In addition to looking at how pain can be modulated at various points along the pathway, this chapter will also cover pain receptors, various neurotransmitters involved in transmitting pain signals to the spinal cord, and pain pathways within the spinal cord. It will highlight the key components of the pathway and elucidate the physiological, cellular, and molecular mechanisms underlying each step.

2.2 Definition

The International Association for the Study of Pain (IASP) defines pain as "an unpleasant sensory and emotional experience associated with actual or potential tissue damage or described in terms of such damage" [1]. Pain perception aims to alert the body's defense system to respond to a stimulus to prevent additional tissue damage.

2.3 Classification of Pain

Pain can be classified based on duration, aetiology, or anatomical location.

2.3.1 Duration

Acute Pain: Short-term pain that is usually associated with tissue injury or inflammation. It serves as an immediate warning system to the body.

Chronic Pain: Pain that persists or recurs for longer than three months is labelled as chronic pain. It refers to the pain that persists beyond the usual time frame for healing and may not be associated with any ongoing tissue damage.

2.3.2 Aetiology

Pain may also be classified as physiological or pathological.

Physiological: Pain that is physiological happens even when there is no real damage to tissues or nerves, and it acts as a signal of potential injury.

Pathological: When pain occurs after tissue damage it's known as pathological pain.

2.3.3 Location

Somatic Pain: Originates from the skin, muscles, bones, or connective tissues. It is often well-localized, such that the individual can typically pinpoint the exact location of the pain.

Visceral Pain: Arises from internal organs such as the stomach, intestines, bladder, or uterus. It is usually less localized and more diffuse than somatic pain, often described as a deep, squeezing, or pressure-like sensation. This type of pain is harder to pinpoint and is frequently associated with an unpleasant, vague discomfort that may be felt over a broader area.

2.4 Initiation, Processing, and Pathway

The peripheral nervous system (PNS) and central nervous system (CNS) mediate all types of pain perception. The primary purpose of the PNS, which is made up of nerves and ganglia outside the brain and spinal cord, is to link the CNS to our body's limbs and organs (Fig. 2.1). The brain and spinal cord make up the CNS, which is primarily in charge of combining and interpreting the data received from the PNS and then coordinating all bodily functions before delivering a response to the effector organs. The events involved in the process are transduction, transmission or conduction, modulation, and perception.

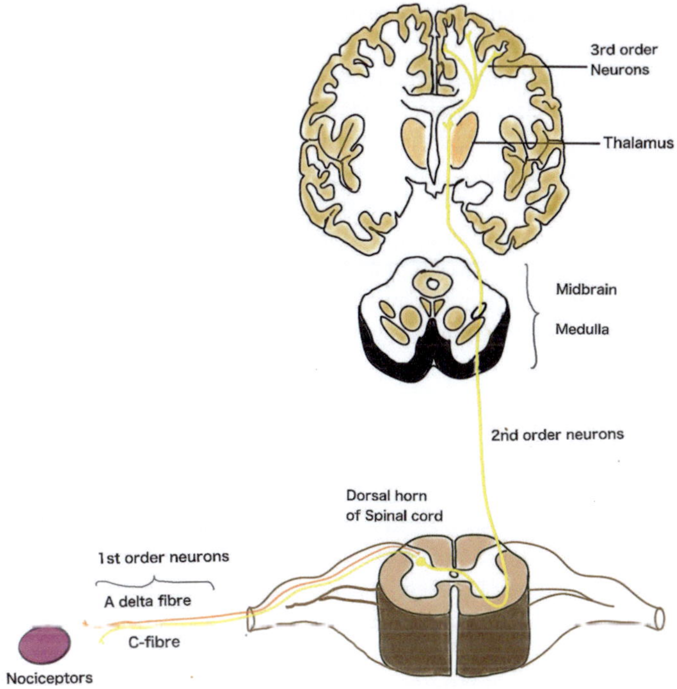

Fig. 2.1 Schematic representation of the pain pathway

2.5 Nociception

The pain pathway begins in the periphery, where specialized sensory receptors are known as nociceptors [2]. These are unencapsulated cutaneous free nerve endings found throughout the body in the skin, joints, muscles, bones, and viscera (internal organs), and they detect potentially harmful stimuli and conduct signals from the periphery to the spinal cord. Every nociceptor possesses a unique receptive field. This indicates that upon stimulation of a specific area of skin, a single nociceptor will transduce the pain signal. Receptive fields vary in size throughout the body and may overlap with adjacent fields.

They are mainly sensitive to three types of noxious stimuli [3, 4]:

1. *Mechanical stimuli:* Sharp objects, pressure, or pinching.
2. *Thermal stimuli:* Extreme temperatures (either heat or cold).
3. *Chemical stimuli:* Inflammatory mediators (e.g., bradykinin, prostaglandins) or irritants (e.g., acid).

The two main functions of the nociceptors are signal transmission (periphery to CNS) and synthetic function (substance P, calcitonin gene-related peptide, and glutamate). The transmission of noxious stimuli is modulated and facilitated by neurotransmitters.

2.5.1 Nociceptors

Nociceptors are specialized sensory receptors responsible for detecting painful stimuli. They play a crucial role in the pain pathway and can be classified based on their morphology, function, and the type of fibers associated with them.

2.5.1.1 Types of Nociceptors

Aδ Fibers

Aδ fibers are a type of nociceptive afferent fiber that play a crucial role in transmitting fast pain signals from peripheral receptors to the CNS. These fibers are myelinated, which allows for faster conduction of nerve impulses compared to unmyelinated fibers (like C fibers). They typically range from 1 to 5 μm in diameter. The conduction velocity is approximately 5 to 30 meters per second, enabling quick transmission of pain signals.

Aδ fibers primarily transmit sharp, localized pain (often referred to as "fast pain") that occurs immediately following an injury. This type of pain is usually well-localized and can be easily pointed out by the person experiencing it. They are also involved in the perception of thermal pain, particularly in response to extreme temperatures. Aδ fibers can be activated by mechanical stimuli like intense pressure or trauma to the skin or thermal stimuli like extreme temperatures (both hot and cold) [5, 6].

Aδ fibers originate from nociceptors located in the skin, muscles, and joints. Thereafter, they enter the spinal cord through the dorsal root and synapse in the dorsal horn, primarily with second-order neurons. Signals are transmitted to the brain via pathways like the spinothalamic tract, reaching areas such as the thalamus and sensory cortex for pain perception [7, 8].

Aδ fibers are crucial in acute pain responses, such as those experienced from cuts or burns. Understanding the function of Aδ fibers helps inform treatment strategies for acute pain relief, such as local anesthetics and certain analgesics.

C Fibers

C fibers are a type of unmyelinated nerve fiber found in the PNS, known for their role in transmitting slow, diffuse pain and other sensory signals. C fibers play a critical role in both acute and chronic pain, serving as the body's way of signaling potential damage and eliciting protective responses. They are thin, with a diameter of 0.2 to 1.5 μm, significantly smaller than myelinated fibers. They conduct impulses at speeds of 0.5 to 2 meters per second, making them the slowest nerve fibers.

C fibers are found in almost all tissues, including skin, muscles, joints, and internal organs, allowing them to sense and report pain from almost any location. C fibers are primarily involved in transmitting dull, aching, and throbbing types of pain. This pain is often poorly localized and can be chronic or persistent, as opposed to the sharp, well-localized pain transmitted by Aδ fibers. They also carry information related to warm temperatures and certain types of itch sensations, especially those triggered by chemical stimuli. Some C fibers, particularly those found in hairy skin, respond to gentle touch and are involved in emotional and social touch.

C fibers are often nociceptive, meaning they respond to noxious (harmful) stimuli that can cause tissue damage. The endings of C fibers act as nociceptors, detecting pain from mechanical, thermal, or chemical damage. Many C fibers are polymodal, meaning they can respond to multiple types of stimuli, including heat, chemical irritants, and tissue injury, making them versatile in the sensation of pain. Chronic stimulation of C fibers can lead to sensitization, where even non-noxious stimuli start to be perceived as painful. This phenomenon is termed as allodynia and is implicated in chronic pain conditions like neuropathic pain and fibromyalgia.

C fibers are integral to the body's pain response, particularly in chronic pain. In conditions of inflammation, these fibers increase their sensitivity, reducing their firing threshold and leading to persistent pain. Factors like tissue acidosis, which lowers the pH at the site of injury, and ATP release from damaged cells stimulate the nociceptive response by activating specific channels on C fibers. Recent studies have shown that thermal changes can significantly enhance these responses, which is why localized heating may worsen the sensation while cooling may temporarily reduce pain [9–11].

Current research is exploring therapeutic strategies that target C-fiber sensitization to manage chronic pain. Modulating TRPV1 and TRPA1 channels, for example, has shown potential in reducing hypersensitivity and may offer relief in chronic pruritus and pain conditions [12, 13].

2.5.2 Neurotransmitters

In pain pathways, neurotransmitters play a crucial role in transmitting pain signals from the site of injury through the spinal cord to the brain. These pathways involve multiple neurotransmitters that either facilitate (excitatory) or inhibit (inhibitory) pain signaling, impacting both acute and chronic pain perception [14–16].

2.5.2.1 Glutamate

It is the primary excitatory neurotransmitter in the pain pathway. It binds to receptors like NMDA, AMPA, etc., on the postsynaptic neurons, leading to an influx of calcium and sodium ions and, thus, neuronal excitation. It plays a prominent role in the transmission of fast, sharp pain signals in the spinal cord's dorsal horn.

Excessive glutamate activity can lead to sensitization and hyperalgesia, contributing to chronic pain. NMDA receptor antagonists (e.g., ketamine) are used in pain management.

2.5.2.2 Substance P

It is an excitatory neuropeptide that amplifies pain signals. It is released by primary afferent fibers in response to painful stimuli and works by binding to neurokinin 1 (NK1) receptors. Substance P facilitates transmission in the dorsal horn and promotes vasodilation and inflammation at injury sites. Its elevated levels are associated with chronic pain conditions like fibromyalgia and arthritis. Hence, NK1 receptor antagonists have been explored as potential pain treatments.

2.5.2.3 Calcitonin Gene-Related Peptide (CGRP)

It's a potent vasodilator and pain transmitter. It is released alongside Substance P from C fibers and binds to CGRP receptors, thus contributing to inflammation and enhancing the perception of pain. It is involved in the transmission of migraine pain and other inflammatory pain conditions.

CGRP antagonists have been developed to block CGRP signaling and to reduce pain in certain headache disorders (e.g., for migraine).

2.5.2.4 GABA (Gamma-Aminobutyric Acid)

It's the primary inhibitory neurotransmitter that dampens pain signaling. It binds to GABA-A and GABA-B receptors, causing an influx of chloride ions and hyperpolarization of the neuron, making it less likely to fire. GABA inhibits nociceptive transmission in the spinal cord's dorsal horn. Low GABA levels are associated with conditions like neuropathic pain.

2.5.2.5 Endorphins and Enkephalins

These are natural opioids that inhibit pain transmission. They bind to opioid receptors (e.g., mu, delta, kappa) on neurons in the brain and spinal cord, inhibiting neurotransmitter release and reducing excitability. They modulate pain perception in the CNS by inhibiting pain signals at various points along the pathway.

Synthetic opioids mimic endorphins to relieve severe pain. However, due to addiction and tolerance risks, they are used cautiously.

2.5.2.6 Norepinephrine

It modulates pain transmission in both excitatory and inhibitory ways depending on receptor types and locations. It activates alpha-2 adrenergic receptors in the dorsal horn, inhibiting the release of excitatory neurotransmitters and reducing pain signals. Additionally, it acts in descending pain pathways originating from the brainstem that help to suppress pain.

Medications like clonidine and dexmedetomidine (alpha-2 adrenergic agonists) use this pathway to treat certain pain types, including neuropathic pain.

2.5.2.7 Serotonin (5-HT)

It's involved in descending pain inhibition and can modulate both inhibitory and excitatory effects. It activates 5-HT receptors in the spinal cord, which can reduce the perception of pain. The descending serotoninergic pathways inhibit nociceptive transmission at the spinal cord level.

Tricyclic antidepressants, which increase serotonin levels, are used to treat certain chronic pain conditions due to serotonin's pain-modulating effects.

2.5.2.8 Dopamine

It modulates pain perception, especially chronic pain. It binds to dopamine receptors, which can modulate pain in the CNS by reducing the intensity of the pain signal. Dopamine pathways in the brain influence pain perception, especially in the limbic system, which processes emotional responses to pain.

Dopamine dysfunction is often seen in chronic pain patients, especially those with fibromyalgia and other central sensitization syndromes.

Table 2.1 summarizes additional neurotransmitters involved in pain pathways, including their roles, mechanisms, and clinical relevance. These neurotransmitters complement primary pain-related neurotransmitters and provide further therapeutic avenues in pain management.

Table 2.1 A summary of additional neurotransmitters which complement primary pain-related neurotransmitters

Neurotransmitter	Role in pain	Mechanism	Clinical relevance
Aspartate	Excitatory neurotransmitter contributing to pain transmission	Binds to NMDA receptors, like glutamate, facilitating neuronal excitation	Often works in conjunction with glutamate in acute and chronic pain; modulating NMDA receptors can aid in pain management
Adenosine	Generally, acts as an inhibitory neuromodulator, reducing pain	Binds to A1 and A2A receptors, which inhibit neurotransmitter release and reduce inflammation	A1 receptor agonists are being explored for neuropathic and inflammatory pain relief
Histamine	Modulates inflammatory pain responses	Binds to H1, H2, H3, and H4 receptors, promoting inflammation and vasodilation	Antihistamines can reduce pain in allergic or inflammatory conditions
Nitric oxide (NO)	Modulates pain sensitization and contributes to chronic pain	Diffuses across membranes, influencing synaptic plasticity and neurotransmitter release, especially glutamate	NO synthesis is linked to central sensitization in chronic pain; NO inhibitors are explored in neuropathic pain management

(continued)

Table 2.1 (continued)

Neurotransmitter	Role in pain	Mechanism	Clinical relevance
Cannabinoids (endocannabinoids)	Reduces pain perception and inflammation	Binds to CB1 and CB2 receptors, modulating neurotransmitter release and inflammatory responses	Cannabis-based treatments target these receptors, effective in certain types of chronic and neuropathic pain
Neurotensin	Modulates pain, with both excitatory and inhibitory effects	Interacts with neurotensin receptors, influencing other neurotransmitter releases	Elevated in inflammatory pain; potential therapeutic target for modulation in chronic pain

A1, *A2A*: Adenosine receptors; *H1*, *H2*, *H3*, and *H4*: Histamine receptors; *CB1*, *CB2*: Cannabinoid receptors; *NMDA*: N-Methyl-D-Aspartate; *NO*: Nitric Oxide

2.6 Physiology of Pain

The process by which a noxious stimulus is perceived as pain by an individual happens in four steps, viz., transduction, transmission, modulation, and perception.

2.6.1 Transduction

The process by which noxious stimuli, such as mechanical, thermal, or chemical injury, are converted into an electrical signal (action potential) by specialized sensory receptors (nociceptors) [17–19]. Following tissue trauma, the affected cells release chemicals (like prostaglandins, bradykinins, and substance P), activating receptors at peripheral axons that convert the stimulus into an electrical signal. These receptors can function alone or in combination to identify and intensify signals produced by noxious stimuli, initiating the electrical impulses sent to the CNS as part of the pain pathway. This process begins by opening transmembrane ion channels on the surface of nociceptor nerve endings, allowing Na^+, K^+, and Cl^- ions to enter the neuron and membrane depolarization. This process is directly proportionated to the intensity of the stimulus [17, 20].

2.6.2 Transmission

Transmission refers to the process by which the electrical signals (action potentials) generated during transduction are transmitted from the site of injury to the brain. The two fibers that transfer pain signals during this process are the Aδ fibers [4, 21, 22], which have a quick and sharp sensation, and the C fibers, which have a delayed sensation. Aδ and C fibers form synapses with neurons in laminas I and V and laminas I and II [23], respectively, in the dorsal horn of the spinal cord, where both fibers terminate. From there, the signals are transmitted through ascending pathways (mainly the spinothalamic tract) to the brain, where pain is perceived. The cells of the dorsal horn are highly malleable, which allows pain impulses to be altered or "gated" there. Different types of neurons occupy a distinct stage in the pathway that relays signals from peripheral tissues to the brain.

2.6.2.1 First-Order Neurons

These neurons carry impulses from the nociceptors to the spinal cord. Their cell bodies are in the dorsal root ganglia of the spinal nerves. Their axons extend from the peripheral sensory receptors to the spinal cord or brainstem.

2.6.2.2 Second-Order Neurons

These neurons serve as a bridge connecting the brainstem and spinal cord to higher brain regions, receiving messages from the first-order neurons. They relay the signal from the spinal cord (or brainstem) to the thalamus, which is the major relay station for sensory information in the brain. Second-order neurons carry on the transmission to the CNS through the two most prominent pathways; the spinothalamic tract and the spinoreticular tract. These tracts often cross over (decussate) to the opposite side of the spinal cord or brainstem before ascending to the thalamus.

Spinothalamic tract is the major pain pathway in humans. Second-order neurons in the dorsal horn send their axons across the midline of the spinal cord and ascend to the brainstem and thalamus, where they synapse with third-order neurons. It has two divisions:

Lateral Spinothalamic Tract: This transmits information for the location, intensity, and quality of pain (the sensory-discriminative aspect).

Anterior Spinothalamic Tract: This transmits information related to the emotional and motivational aspects of pain.

The spinoreticular tract is involved in the emotional and arousal aspects of pain. Signals from the spinoreticular tract project to the reticular formation in the brainstem, which then sends signals to the thalamus and other brain regions involved in emotional responses.

Additionally, the spinomesencephalic tract carries pain signals to the periaqueductal gray (PAG) in the midbrain, where descending pain control mechanisms are initiated. This pathway plays a crucial role in pain modulation and the release of endogenous opioids.

2.6.2.3 Third-Order Neurons

These transmit the sensory information from the thalamus to the appropriate region of the cerebral cortex, where the signal is finally processed and interpreted. Third-order neurons relay the signal from the thalamus to the primary somatosensory cortex in the parietal lobe of the brain. The cell bodies of third-order neurons are in the thalamus. Their axons project to specific areas of the cortex, where the sensory information is perceived, localized, and understood (e.g., pain, temperature, touch). The perception, location, and emotional aspects of pain are mediated by third-order neurons in the thalamus.

2.6.3 Modulation

The process by which the body modifies a pain signal as it travels along the pain pathway is known as pain modulation, and it helps to explain why different people may react differently to the same painful stimuli. Pain modulation can occur at multiple levels within the nervous system, particularly in the spinal cord and brain. It involves several pathways, neurotransmitters, and endogenous (natural) substances that can either enhance (facilitate) or suppress (inhibit) pain signals.

2.6.3.1 Descending Pain Modulation

Descending modulation refers to the brain's ability to influence pain perception by sending signals down the spinal cord to either inhibit or enhance pain. Two crucial brain regions involved in descending inhibitory regulation are the rostral ventromedial medulla (RVM) and the periaqueductal grey (PAG) in the midbrain [24, 25]. High levels of endogenous opioids and opioid receptors are found in both locations, which explains the analgesic properties of opioids. Activation of PAG leads to the release of inhibitory neurotransmitters (such as serotonin and norepinephrine) to reduce the intensity of the pain signal.

2.6.3.2 Ascending Pain Modulation

Ascending pathways transmit pain signals from the site of injury to the brain. However, pain signals can be modulated in the spinal cord before they reach higher centers. This modulation primarily occurs at the level of the dorsal horn of the spinal cord, where sensory neurons synapse. One of the most well-known mechanisms of pain modulation at the spinal level is the gate control theory, proposed by Melzack and Wall in 1965 [26–28]. This theory suggests that a non-painful stimulus can "close the gate" to painful stimuli by activating inhibitory interneurons in the dorsal horn. For example, rubbing a painful area can help reduce the sensation of pain by activating touch receptors that inhibit nociceptive signals.

2.6.4 Perception

Both the sensory and emotional aspects of pain are processed by several interrelated brain regions, making pain perception a multifaceted and intricate experience. When nociceptors, or specialized pain receptors, detect painful stimuli, signals are sent to the spinal cord via peripheral nerves. Information from third-order neurons that go to the cerebral cortex is mostly processed in the thalamus. The thalamus acts as a sensory relay station, directing pain signals to different parts of the brain for processing [29]. It plays a pivotal role in the perception of pain, particularly its location, intensity, and duration. Somatosensory cortex, anterior cingulate cortex (ACC), insula, prefrontal cortex, amygdala are the primary brain areas involved in pain perception [30].

2.7 Peripheral Sensitization

Peripheral sensitization occurs when nerve endings in the PNS become more sensitive to stimuli following an injury or inflammation. This heightened sensitivity results from chemical changes around the damaged or inflamed area. When tissue is injured or inflamed, cells release chemicals like prostaglandins, histamine, bradykinin, and cytokines. These chemicals activate and increase the sensitivity of nociceptors in the area. This process lowers the activation threshold of the nociceptors, meaning even light touches or mild heat, which would typically not cause pain, can trigger a pain response.

2.8 Central Sensitization

Central sensitization occurs when neurons in the CNS become hypersensitive. This increased sensitivity makes pain signals stronger and more widespread, and it can persist even after the original injury or inflammation has healed. Central sensitization is a significant contributor to chronic pain syndromes, such as fibromyalgia, migraines, and chronic low back pain. In central sensitization, prolonged pain signaling from the PNS causes structural and functional changes in the CNS. These changes lower the threshold for pain and amplify the response to pain signals, causing normal sensations to feel painful (allodynia) and painful sensations to feel worse than they would otherwise (hyperalgesia).

2.9 Hyperalgesia

It is a phenomenon where there is an exaggerated response to painful stimuli, meaning a stimulus that would typically cause mild pain results in an unusually intense pain experience. This heightened sensitivity can result from both peripheral and central mechanisms and is commonly associated with chronic pain conditions.

2.10 Allodynia

It is a condition in which a person experiences pain from stimuli that would not normally be painful. For instance, a gentle touch, brushing of the skin, or even a light breeze can cause pain in individuals with allodynia. It is commonly associated with conditions involving chronic pain.

2.11 Conclusion

The pain pathway is a complex and highly coordinated system that involves multiple layers of sensory processing and modulation, from peripheral nociceptors detecting harmful stimuli to the brain interpreting these signals as pain. This pathway not only allows us to respond to injury and protect ourselves but also provides opportunities for therapeutic intervention in cases of chronic or pathological pain. By understanding the mechanisms underlying pain transmission and perception, clinicians and researchers can develop more effective treatments for managing pain and improving quality of life.

Acknowledgments We acknowledge the contribution of Dr. Nehal Singh in digitally drawing the Fig. 2.1.

References

1. IASP. IASP terminology. 2017. Available at: https://www.iasp-pain.org/Education/Content.aspx?ItemNumber5 1698.
2. Ballantyne JC, Fishman SM, Rathmell JP. Bonica's management of pain. 5th ed. Lippincott Williams & Wilkins; 2018. p. 11–34.
3. Sneddon LU. Comparative physiology of nociception and pain. Physiology (Bethesda). 2018;33(1):63–73.
4. Yam MF, Loh YC, Tan CS, et al. General pathways of pain sensation and the major neurotransmitters involved in pain regulation. Int J Mol Sci. 2018;19(8):1–23.
5. Vincent W, Yam J, Berger M. Developmental changes in DRG neurons: implications for pain perception. J Clin Invest. 2020;130(9):4516–23.
6. Avraham O, Harty BL, Monk KR. Satellite glial cells in pain signaling. Front Cell Neurosci. 2022;16:778344.
7. Nascimento R, Vincent M. Mechanisms of nociceptor response to thermal stimuli. J Pain Res. 2018;11:347–54.
8. Giovannini T, et al. Emerging axonal signaling in neuropathic pain: DRG neuron plasticity. Pain Med. 2021:21(S1).
9. Hashimoto S, Tanaka Y. Brain-derived neurotrophic factor and nociceptive sensitization. Curr Neuropharmacol. 2013;11(6):570–5.
10. Casimir CM, Barrette JH, Kallurkar M, Levine JD. The contribution of C-fiber sensory neurons to nociceptive behavior. Pain Rep. 2018;3(4)
11. Dosch M, Ingle A, Sopko N, Mitchell SR. Molecular mechanisms and contributions of the TRPV1 channel in neurogenic inflammation and pain pathways. Front Mol Neurosci. 2018;11:275.
12. Villalba-Riquelme E, Gonzalez-Pina R, Villeda-Hernandez J, Aceves-Martins M, Montoya-Alvarez V, Torres-Perez M, Quintanar-Stephano A. Chronic pain and pruritus in the skin: role of TRPV1 channels. Front Pharmacol. 2022;13:846932.
13. Bagood MD, Isseroff RR. TRPV1 as a therapeutic target for pruritus and pain: soft modulation in the skin. Front Pharmacol. 2021;12:737689.
14. Tan CS, Adam SK, Manan NA, Basir R. General pathways of pain sensation and the major neurotransmitters involved in pain regulation. Int J Mol Sci. 2018;19(8):2164.
15. Gupta R, Harvima IT. Neuroinflammatory mechanisms in chronic pain. Front Cell Neurosci. 2018;12:1–15.
16. Wang Y, Nakai T, Inoue K. Serotonergic and GABAergic modulation in chronic pain. J Pain Res. 2021;14:456–67.

17. Devor M. Neurobiology of normal and pathophysiologic pain. In: Aranoff GM, editor. Evaluation and treatment of chronic pain. 3rd ed. Philadelphia: Lippincott Williams & Wilkins; 1999. p. 11–25.
18. Katz N, Ferrante FM. Nociception. In: Ferrante FM, VadeBoncouer TR, editors. Postop erative pain management. New York: Churchill Livingstone; 1993. p. 17–67.
19. Suchdev PK. Pathophysiologyofpain. In: Warfield, Fausett HJ, editors. Manualofpain management. Philadelphia: Lippincott Williams & Wilkins; 2002. p. 6–12.
20. Byers MR, Bonica JJ. Peripheral pain mechanisms and nociceptor plasticity. In: Loeser JD, editor. Bonica's management of pain. 3rd ed. Philadelphia: Lippincott Williams & Wilkins; 2001. p. 26–72.
21. Lin ES. Physiology of pain. In: Smith T, Pinnock C, Lin T, editors. Fundamentals of anaesthesia. 3rd ed. Cambridge: Cambridge University Press; 2009. p. 412–32.
22. Coda BA, Bonica JJ. General considerations of acute pain. In: Loeser JD, editor. Bonica's management of pain. 3rd ed. Philadelphia: Lippincott Williams & Wilkins; 2001. p. 222–40.
23. Dubin AE, Patapoutian A. Nociceptors: the sensors of the pain pathway. J Clin Invest. 2010;120:3760–72.
24. Freund W, Wunderlich AP, Stuber G, et al. The role of the periaqueductal gray and cingulate cortex during suppression of pain in complex regional pain syndrome. Clin J Pain. 2011;27:796–804.
25. Mokhtar M, Singh P, Neuroanatomy, Periaqueductal Gray. StatPearls. Treasure Island: StatPearls Publishing; 2021. p. 2022.
26. Melzack R, Wall PD. Pain mechanisms: a new theory. Science. 1965;150(3699):971–9.
27. Wall PD, Melzack R. Textbook of pain. Edinburgh: Churchill Livingstone; 1994.
28. Jensen MP, Brownstone RM. Mechanisms of spinal cord stimulation for the treatment of pain: still in the dark after 50 years. Eur J Pain. 2019;23:652–9.
29. Vrooman BM, Youngren KM. Chronic pain management. In: Butterworth IV JF, Mackey DC, Wasnick JD, editors. Morgan and Mikhail's clinical anesthesiology. 7th ed. McGraw Hill; 2022. p. 1071–82.
30. Isa AS, Chetty S. Physiology and pathophysiology of chronic pain (part I). South Afr J Anaesth Analg. 2021;27(6):266–70.

Pre-emptive or Preventive Analgesia

3

Pallavi Ahluwalia and Kumari Tripta

Abstract

Preventing or minimizing central nervous system sensitivity and sensory disruptions during surgery, extending the duration of pain relief, and minimizing the use of analgesics are the best ways to manage postoperative pain. Taking effective measures to relieve pain in advance and reduce the pain sensitivity of central and peripheral nerves before harmful stimulation by surgery can accelerate the recovery of patients and significantly reduce the patient's surgical trauma and postoperative pain compared with analgesia given after the start of pain. The intervention of central neuraxial sensitization and peripheral sensitization to stop the spread of pain and achieve postoperative pain relief is known as preemptive analgesia (PA). PA has emerged as a popular therapeutic approach for anesthesiologists treating postoperative patient-controlled analgesia. Clinical guidelines for advanced analgesia are still missing, though.

P. Ahluwalia (✉) · K. Tripta
Department of Anaesthesiology, Teerthanker Mahaveer Medical College (TMMC), Moradabad, Uttar Pradesh, India

P. Ahluwalia (ed.), *Handbook of Perioperative Analgesia*,
https://doi.org/10.1007/978-981-96-7822-8_3

Keywords

Preventive analgesia · Central sensitization · Hyperalgesia · Chronic post-surgical pain (CPSP)

Key Points

- Preventive analgesia reduces perioperative pain by inhibiting central and peripheral sensitization.
- Central sensitization is a complex process that occurs due to an increase in membrane excitability in response to noxious stimuli of surgery.
- The main aim of preventive analgesia is to reduce acute pain, prevent chronic pain, reduce the need for analgesic drugs, and decrease hospital stay after surgery.
- The best intervention for preventive analgesia is to use a combination of different modalities that act on different pain receptors.
- The plan for analgesia is based on the type of surgery, duration of surgery, patient factor, and best route of drug administration.

3.1 Introduction

The concept of pre-emptive analgesia (PA) was first introduced by "Crile" in the early twentieth century and refers to the reduction of postoperative pain by administering analgesics before surgical incision [1]. Acute postoperative pain is the result of tissue injury to neuronal or visceral structures during surgical procedures. The idea of PA for the treatment of acute pain was based on experiments based on the hypothesis that preventing access to noxious stimuli to the central nervous system (CNS) is more beneficial than administering analgesics after surgery [2]. It has been estimated that acute postoperative pain is followed by persistent pain in 10–50% of patients and that it may be severe in approximately 2–10% of these patients [3]. Therefore, persistent postoperative pain has increasingly come into focus in recent years.

The main reason for persistent pain is unrelieved severe perioperative pain, which can be reduced by aggressive preventive methods such as analgesics, nerve blocks, and multimodal analgesia. The terms "pre-emptive" and "PA" are used interchangeably and there is confusion and controversy regarding the terminology. Preventive analgesia refers to any procedure before the incision that prevents the development of central sensitization due to incisional and inflammatory injuries [4]. "Preventive" analgesia assumes that the only way to prevent central sensitization is to completely block all pain signals from the surgical wound from the time of skin incision until final wound healing [5]. Preventive analgesia focuses on the intensity and duration of analgesic treatment [6]. The term "preventive analgesia" is now considered a more appropriate term as it includes all perioperative measures performed during the perioperative period to relieve postoperative pain and reduce the consumption of analgesics [7] (Fig. 3.1).

Several unique factors can contribute to postoperative pain, including preoperative traumatic stimulation and pre-existing pain, intraoperative surgical incisions, postoperative inflammatory response, and ectopic neuron activation. Therefore, minimizing the impact of factors that aid in inhibiting peripheral and

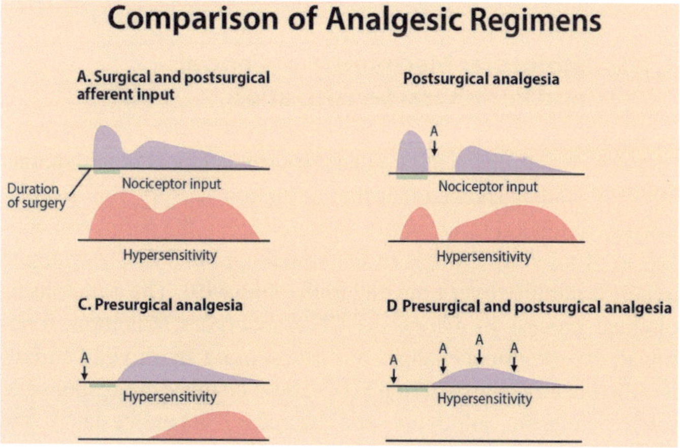

Fig. 3.1 The concept of preventive analgesia

central sensitization in the three stages of sensitization and preventing the transmission of pain signals from tissue damage to wound healing are the best approaches.

Initially, there's a phase focused on pain perception, then comes the second phase where impulses are relayed from the outermost regions to the dorsal horn (DH), situated within the spinal cord, through the peripheral nervous system (PNS). Ultimately, the third phase involves transmitting these signals to the superior brain regions using the central nervous system (CNS). In addition, the surgical procedure, magnitude, duration, operation time, analgesic methods, and the nature of analgesic drugs before the tissue injury will also affect the degree of pain after the operation. Conduction of pain from the periphery to the center is a complex process and depends on the balance between excitatory and inhibitory systems. One or several stages of pain transmission can be blocked to prevent peripheral and central hypersensitivity. The use of PA reduces postoperative pain, opioid consumption, and postoperative nausea or vomiting, and delays rescue analgesia [8]. After the concept of PA gained widespread acceptance, the benefits of PA in relieving postoperative pain and reducing analgesic consumption received clinical and research attention for many years.

3.1.1 Molecular Mechanism of Central and Peripheral Sensitization

In 1989, Woolf and King coined the term "central sensitization" after the studies showed that the motor and sensory changes following peripheral tissue injury were related to the peripheral activation of afferent C fibers in the spinal cord and they developed hyperexcitability over time due to the injury [9]. The pathophysiological process by which the CNS undergoes structural, functional, and chemical changes to make it more sensitive to stimuli is called central sensitization [10]. These changes are responsible for hyperalgesia, allodynia, and secondary hyperalgesia. A few terminologies, commonly used, are listed below:

- Hyperalgesia: It is a condition in which a person experiences increased pain sensitivity.
- Allodynia: Pain is felt due to a stimulus that does not normally cause pain, such as touch.
- Secondary hyperalgesia: There is increased sensitivity to mechanical pain in areas not directly affected by injury.

3.1.2 Peripheral Sensitization

The establishment of sensitization in the periphery involves the transition from high-threshold nociceptors to low-threshold nociceptors, which is induced by the release of various chemicals shortly after surgical incision. A complex array of inflammatory mediators arises at the site of damage and are mobilized from injured tissue, while others are delivered via the circulation. Small-diameter primary afferent neurons, Aδ and C fibers, which innervate the region of injury, subsequently enter a state that is characterized by sustained discharge, a lowered activation threshold, and excitation induced by supra-threshold stimulation (hyperalgesia). The center of a surgical wound, which is the primary zone of injury, is expected to exhibit static mechanical hyperalgesia [11] (Fig. 3.2).

The following factors play an important role in peripheral sensitization, as listed below:

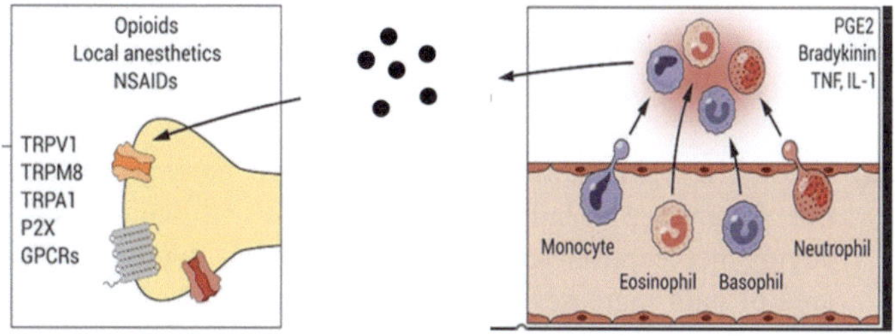

Fig. 3.2 Peripheral sensitization during inflammation

(a) Upregulation of active nociceptors.
(b) Sensitization of the primary afferent terminals.
(c) Generation of ectopic discharges as a result of increased sodium and calcium channel activity.
(d) Phenotype switching results in increased production of excitatory neuropeptides like substance P, CGRP, etc.
(e) Somatic-sympathetic coupling: Catecholamines bind and stimulate sensitized nociceptors to generate an action potential.

3.1.3 Central Sensitization

The molecular mechanism of central sensitization is a complex process involving an early, nociceptor-driven response. Nociplastic pain, previously known as central sensitisation is due to an increase in membrane excitability, synaptic efficacy, and reduced inhibition of somatosensory and nociceptive pathways in response to nociception, inflammation, and nerve damage [12]. Tissue injuries release chemicals such as leukotrienes and potassium. Platelets release serotonin and vascular injury results in the release of bradykinin from plasma, leading to the activation of nociceptors [13, 14]. This activation causes the release of nociceptive signals via the nociceptors of the A and C fibers to the dorsal horn of the spinal cord, which in turn release neurotransmitters such as excitatory amino acids, glutamate, and aspartate, as well as substances such as substance P and calcitonin gene-related peptide, which increase the responses of the dorsal horn neurons, resulting in central sensitization [15].

The following factors are components of central sensitization:

(a) Central reorganization—Following nerve damage, A beta fibers converge in lamina II and synapse with neurons conveying nociception resulting in mechanical allodynia. The area of pain increases along the distribution of other nerves due to the activation of interneurons at the spinal level. There is a loss of function of descending inhibitory pathways.

(b) Disinhibition—Downregulation of GABA, glycine, and opioid receptors in the dorsal horn of the spinal cord.
(c) Ectopic discharges.
(d) Windup phenomena—Repeated stimulation of C fibers results in temporal summation of inputs and results in an increase in the excitatory stimulus.
(e) Activation of wide dynamic range neurons [16].

3.1.4 Mechanisms of Acute Versus Chronic Pain

In the past, there have been two major models of pain. The first stated that there are specific pain pathways that are activated by peripheral pain stimuli and that the intensity and duration of pain depend only on the input. Acute pain was considered a protective phenomenon against noxious stimuli that activated a peripheral nerve that sent signals to the brain via the spinal cord. But now we know that this process is more complicated and that these stimuli are received neurochemically, signals are amplified or inhibited in the brain, and the modulated messages are sent back through special neural pathways [17]. The second model is the "gate control theory" which suggests that substantia gelatinosa in dorsal horn of spinal cord acts as a gate and modulates transmission of pain signals to the brain. For example, in chronic pain, neuroplasticity makes nerves more sensitive to stimulation, and pain signaling is not just a protective response to noxious stimuli. Rather, pain signals are a result of maladaptive changes in the nervous system and not necessarily a response to acute nociceptive stimuli [18].

3.2 Preoperative Preparation

Patients undergoing minor or major surgery are prone to postoperative pain. The problem of inadequate postoperative pain control can lead to adverse physiological effects in the immediate postoperative period. There is an increased risk of developing chronic pain related to the procedure. Therefore, for effective management of postoperative pain, the anesthesiologist must have a well-formulated and patient-centric perioperative pain management strategy. Before any procedure, it is prudent to review the patient's medical history; to identify the risk factors and comorbidities that may influence the severity of postoperative pain. Careful pain management should consider the type of procedure, previous pain reactions, previous exposure to pain medications, current medications, fears or concerns about future pain, and history of chronic opioid use. It has also been reported in the literature that patients who underwent major spinal, orthopedic, or traumatic extremity surgeries had higher postoperative pain scores [19]. Preoperative opioid use and dependence have also been found to be associated with greater postoperative pain levels and increased opioid requirements (discussed separately in Chap. 7). Preoperative psychological factors such as catastrophism, depression, anxiety, and pain expectancy are also important predictors of high postoperative acute pain intensity.

3.3 Chronic Postsurgical Pain (CPSP)

Chronic postsurgical pain (CPSP) was first defined by Macrae and Davies [20] in 1999 and later expanded by Macrae in 2001 [21] and refers to pain after any surgical procedure lasting at least 2 months, with all other causes of pain excluded. The updated definition proposed by Werner and Kongsgaard in 2014 "pain that is localized to the surgical site or a referred area, lasts for at least three months following surgery, was absent before surgery, or differs from preoperative pain in terms of its characteristics or intensity" [22]. Inflammatory processes or the triggering of neuropathic pain by peripheral nerve damage during surgery leads to severe tissue damage. The incidence of CPSP varies between different surgeries, ranging from 5% to 85% [23]. There is no definitive way to prevent it, but it is generally accepted that multimodal analgesia, recognition of the risk factor, and the use of minimally invasive surgical procedures (that avoid nerve damage) help prevent long-term postoperative pain. Risk factors for CPSP include approach and type of surgery, patient factors such as women being more susceptible, young adults, genetic predisposition, and psychosocial factors (Fig. 3.3).

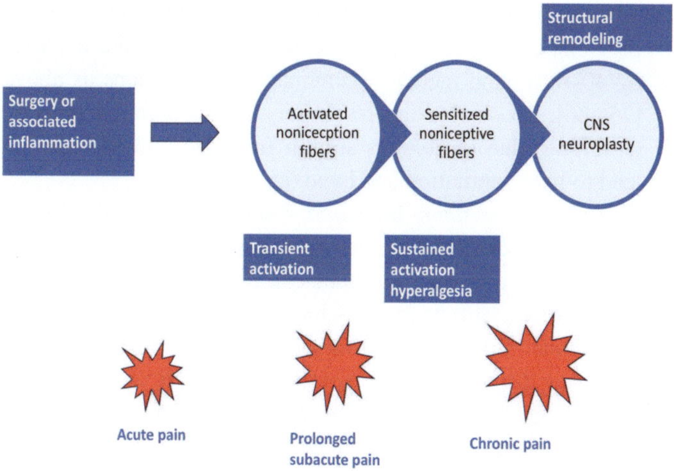

Fig. 3.3 Chronic post-surgical pain development

3.4 Adverse Effect of Postsurgical Pain

Unrelieved postoperative pain results in physical, cognitive, and emotional discomfort, leading to significant morbidity and mortality. It can also lead to delayed recovery, longer hospital stays, greater utilization of healthcare resources, and higher healthcare costs. Anger and resentment can be expressed as a result of ongoing, unrelieved sorrow. Patients become depressed and helpless as a result of losing control over their surroundings.

3.4.1 Physiological Consequences of Unrelieved Pain

Cardiovascular system: The overactivity of the autonomic nervous system brought on by pain leads to sympathetic activation, which raises the cardiac workload, raises the myocardial oxygen demand, and lowers the myocardial oxygen supply. Myocardial ischemia, angina, and myocardial infarction may result from this [24].

Respiratory system: Pain after thoracic and upper abdominal surgery can cause pulmonary dysfunction, reduce vital capacity by 40–60%, and increase pulmonary complications as above [25, 26]. Spasms of the respiratory and abdominal muscles (splinting) due to noxious stimuli from the injured area can lead to hypoventilation and hypoxia.

Gastrointestinal system: Increased sympathetic activity due to severe pain can lead to increased gastrointestinal secretion, increased smooth muscle sphincter tone, and decreased intestinal motility, resulting in ileus, nausea, and vomiting.

Coagulation: Surgical stress triggers a metabolic response that increases thromboembolism, venostasis, deep vein thrombosis, and platelet aggregation. This is further worsened by immobilization brought on by insufficient pain management.

Renal system: Urinary sphincter tone is increased, bladder tone is inhibited, and urine retention occurs as a result of the surgical response's enhanced sympathetic activity.

3.5 Prevention of Postoperative Pain by Preventive Analgesia

Preventive analgesia includes multimodal interventions to reduce nociceptive stimuli. It is started preoperatively and extended to the postoperative period. It helps relieve postoperative pain and reduces unwanted side effects, allowing for faster recovery and earlier hospital discharge [27].

To formulate an effective plan for preventive analgesia, several critical factors must be carefully considered to ensure optimal pain management. These factors span the procedure itself, the patient's characteristics, and the pharmacological tools available, along with an ongoing assessment strategy to ensure effectiveness. The following elements must be addressed:

- *Type of procedure*—It plays a significant role in determining the approach to analgesia. Different surgical procedures generate varying levels of pain. For instance, major surgeries such as open abdominal procedures or orthopedic surgeries may require more aggressive pain management strategies compared to minor procedures like laparoscopic surgeries or superficial excisions.

- *Location, duration, and intensity of injury*—The location of the injury or surgical site is important, as pain from certain anatomical regions (such as the abdomen or thorax) can be more intense and complex compared to others (such as superficial wounds). The duration of the injury or procedure will influence the need for longer-acting or extended-release analgesics. The intensity of injury also plays a crucial role. For example, trauma to highly innervated areas may require more intensive pain control compared to less sensitive regions.
- *Patient characteristics*—Patient personality or behavior can impact how they experience and report pain. Some patients may have heightened pain sensitivity or a low pain tolerance, necessitating a more individualized approach to analgesia.
- *Pre-existing comorbidities* (such as diabetes, hypertension, or renal dysfunction) must be considered when choosing analgesics, as certain drugs may be contraindicated or require dose adjustments based on the patient's overall health.
- The *postoperative course* is a key consideration. For patients who are likely to require an intensive care unit (ICU) stay, continuous or more potent analgesia may be necessary to ensure comfort and minimize stress response. Conversely, those on the ward may be better managed with oral medications or less aggressive intravenous (IV) options.
- Whether the patient is intubated or extubated is another important factor, as intubated patients often require deeper levels of sedation and analgesia to ensure comfort and prevent awareness during mechanical ventilation.
- *Pharmacological options available*—There is a wide range of pharmacological agents available for preventive analgesia, and the choice of drug depends on the procedure, patient factors, and potential for side effects. These options include opioids, non-opioid analgesics, NSAIDs, and local anesthetics. For example, IV opioids may be needed in the immediate postop-

erative period, while oral analgesics can be used for sustained pain relief once the patient is stable.

- *Methods of drug administration*—Continuous infusion, intermittent bolus, or patient-controlled analgesia (PCA) are different methods of drug delivery. The method selected should reflect both the pain intensity and the patient's ability to manage analgesia.

3.6 Interventions for Preventive Analgesia

Different treatment modalities can be practiced. Preventive analgesics can be used individually or in combination. However, regional anesthesia and intravenous opioids have been studied more extensively and found to be more beneficial. Other options include nonsteroidal anti-inflammatory drugs (NSAIDs), N-methyl-D-aspartate (NMDA) receptor antagonists, nerve blocks, neuraxial local anesthetics, neuraxial opioids, intravenous or epidural ketamine, and lidocaine.

3.6.1 Regional Anesthesia

Various neuraxial and peripheral regional techniques can be used. These are site-specific, superior to systemic opioids, and reduce mortality and morbidity [28].

(a) *Single-dose neuraxial opioids*
Opioids can be administered directly in the subarachnoid space or into the epidural space. The hydrophilic opioid (morphine or hydromorphone) has a delayed onset and longer duration of action. It has a common side effect due to supraspinal spread. Lipophilic opioids such as (fentanyl and sufentanil) have a rapid onset and shorter duration of action but may cause delayed respiratory depression. Depending on the type of surgery and the patient's profile, either lipophilic or hydrophilic opioids can be administered as a single dose

intrathecally or epidurally. When the epidural catheter's position is not near the surgical incision, a single dosage of hydrophilic opioids is very beneficial for postoperative epidural analgesia.

(b) *Continuous Epidural Analgesia (CEA)*
Epidural infusion of local anesthetics has a higher incidence of hypotension so they are used with adjuvants such as opioids [29]. Continuous epidural anesthesia is not commonly used for PA. However, one study by Farouk showed that continuous epidural magnesium, when started before anesthesia, can offer PA and an analgesic-sparing effect without increasing side effects [30].

(c) *Patient-Controlled Epidural Analgesia (PCEA)*
In addition to offering better analgesia than intravenous patient-controlled analgesia (IV PCA), PCEA has benefits over CEA, including reduced analgesic requirements and increased patient satisfaction. Low concentrations of local anesthetics mixed with opioids work better together to control pain than they do separately.

(d) *Peripheral Regional Blocks*
This can give site-specific analgesia and can be administered as a single injection or as a continuous infusion. Peripheral blocks have several advantages over neuraxial blocks, such as a lower risk of spinal hematoma and less hemodynamic instability. They can be given to patients with hemodynamic instability or patients with abnormalities in hemostasis or infection. The duration and quality of nerve blocks can be prolonged with adjuvants such as dexamethasone, clonidine, or dexmedetomidine, etc. Continuous infusion via a peripheral nerve catheter facilitates early postoperative rehabilitation, shortens hospital stay, and increases mobility. Paravertebral block and thoracic epidural provide the same analgesic effect, but paravertebral block has a better safety profile in terms of less hypotension although pneumothorax remains a potential complication. Continuous infusions provide better pain control than intermittent doses [31].

3.6.2 Intra-articular and Local Infiltration Analgesia

Up to 72 h following high-volume local anesthetic infiltration, patients undergoing total knee arthroplasty (TKR) and total hip arthroplasty (THR) had lower pain levels and opioid needs, according to a systemic study [32]. A brief period of postoperative analgesia is provided by intra-articular injection of NSAID and local analgesia. The peripheral end of the principal efferent nerves contains peripheral opioid receptors. Following local opioid delivery, these receptors provide postoperative analgesia because they are increased during inflammation. Nevertheless, some research indicates that morphine injected intra-articularly following knee surgery has no analgesic effect [33].

3.6.3 Systemic Analgesics

3.6.3.1 Opioids

Compared to regional analgesia, there are fewer studies on preventative opioid analgesia. Opioids can be administered either intramuscularly, subcutaneously, transcutaneous, or transmucosal, but are most commonly administered as intravenous drugs or orally because of their rapid and reliable onset of action. However, the limitation of opioids is the development of tolerance and side effects such as nausea, vomiting, and shortness of breath. Overall, despite this limitation, the evidence for the effectiveness of opioids is positive. Systemic opioids along with regional opioids are effective in various preventive analgesia studies. A single intervention with short-acting opioids such as alfentanil, remifentanil, or fentanyl is not effective for preventive analgesia because it allows a window period for central sensitization. Opioids are more potent and longer-acting than NSAIDs. Their prolonged use can lead to tolerance, dependence, withdrawal, and even nociceptive sensitization reactions, which can increase pain, and, therefore, it is challenging for medical professionals to successfully manage patients' pain, and develop safe and efficient analgesic techniques.

3.6.4 NSAIDS and COX Inhibitors

By blocking cyclooxygenase (COX) and influencing prostaglandin synthesis, non-steroidal anti-inflammatory medications (NSAIDs) have analgesic and antipyretic effects. Maintaining and extending the analgesic effect till the postoperative inflammatory phase is the aim of NSAIDS in preventive analgesia. Inhibiting co-oxygenase and prostaglandin synthesis, which mediates hyperalgesia and peripheral sensitization and may also inhibit spinal COX, is the main way that NSAIDs work [34]. Inhibition of spinal PGE2 production by NSAIDs that inhibit COX2 appears to be the primary mechanism of preventive hyperalgesia in animal models. The mainstay of preventive analgesia is timing, an effective analgesic regime given before the onset of noxious stimuli. A meta-analysis done by Ochroch et al. demonstrates that the NSAIDs used currently for preventive analgesia alone do not provide significant perioperative pain reduction in the long term but they will play a major role in multimodal analgesia and pain relief in general [35]. A recent meta-analysis evaluating the effects of perioperative NSAIDs during spinal fusion revealed that high-dose ketorolac improved outcomes in adults undergoing spinal fusion surgery [36]. In individuals with normal perioperative renal function, the use of NSAIDs during surgery is unlikely to have an impact on renal function. However, they may have deleterious effects in patients with hypovolemia, and abnormal serum electrolyte or renal function, as prostaglandins (inhibited by NSAIDs) mediate diuretic and natriuretic effects through vasodilatation. As compared to traditional NSAIDs, selective COX-2 inhibitors provide analgesia with fewer side effects. Long-term use of COX-2 inhibitors carries a high cardiovascular risk, which depends on many factors such as the specific drug, dosage, or patient characteristics. The use of a strong COX2 inhibitor (Rofecoxib) in high cardiac risk cases (bypass surgery) results in a higher rate of cardiovascular events compared to non-cardiac cases [37]. Administration of NSAIDs alone provides effective analgesia, but cannot provide effective analgesia before surgical incision. Therefore, NSAIDs alone do not meet the criteria for preventive analgesia.

3.6.5 Acetaminophen

It contains anti-inflammatory and antipyretic qualities. Additionally, it has a central analgesic action that is mediated by the brain's descending serotonergic pathway being activated. This could be because it inhibits the creation of prostaglandins or because it contains an active metabolite that affects cannabinoid receptors. It is mostly used as a multimodal analgesia together with other medications. Acetaminophen is a widely used non-opioid drug for managing pain and fever with a better safety profile. However, the optimal timing for acetaminophen administration for pain control is not well defined several studies have shown the administration of acetaminophen is effective as preventive analgesia [38, 39]. It inhibits many of the enzymes in the inflammatory pathways, including COX1, COX2, and myeloperoxidases [40].

3.6.6 NMDA Receptor Antagonist

NMDA receptor antagonists such as ketamine prevent central neuroplasticity and therefore play a role in preventative analgesia by reducing central sensitization. Ketamine is an analgesic that can be given orally, intravenously (PCA or continuous infusion), subcutaneously, or intramuscularly. It may be crucial in reducing opioid tolerance and central sensitization. The limitation of perioperative use of ketamine infusion is an amnestic effect at the cognitive and neuropharmacological levels. Ketamine can also be administered epidurally or intrathecally, but a racemic mixture is avoided due to its neurotoxic nature. The dose ranges from 0.2 to 0.5 mg/kg IV bolus and 0.06 to 0.6 mg/kg/h continuous infusion. Larger doses can cause respiratory depression. Small doses of an anti-sialagogue may be necessary to prevent excessive salivation. At higher doses, dissociative states can be induced by the disconnection of the thalamocortical and limbic systems [41]. Subramaniam et al. studied the use of ketamine via the epidural route in 46 ASA physical status I and II patients who underwent major upper abdominal surgery [42]. They found that in patients undergoing major abdominal surgery there was improved analgesia without the increase of side effects during administration of dilute epidural ketamine at a dose of 1 mg/kg with morphine 50 μg/kg. Dextromethorphan is an NMDA receptor antagonist. This drug acts similarly to ketamine but has less affinity to the NMDA receptors. It can help reduce neuropathic pain and enhance the analgesic impact of morphine on acute pain following surgery [43].

3.6.7 Gabapentinoids

The multimodal analgesia paradigm makes use of gabapentinoids, including pregabalin and gabapentin. This class of antiepileptic medications works by blocking the calcium channel, which prevents calcium from entering the body and excitatory neurotransmitters from being released. Neuropathic pain is treated using them. Recent studies suggest that gabapentin may have minimal opioid effects, but the incidence of adverse effects is increasing during laparoscopic procedures and gabapentin use is associated with respiratory distress [44]. Hence, the use of gabapentinoids should be considered on an individual basis after surgery. According to a recent systematic review. Gabapentin and COX-2 inhibitors were found to be the most effective pre-emptive analgesics for postoperative pain control [45].

Gamma-aminobutyric acid's structural counterpart is gabapentin. It has antinociceptive, antihyperalgesic, and antiallodynic effects by attaching itself to the α2-δ protein subunit of presynaptic voltage-gated calcium channels in the central and peripheral nervous systems [46].

Pregabalin has a better pharmacological and pharmacokinetic profile than gamma-aminobutyric acid, despite being a structural homolog [47]. It is a stronger and more efficient gabapentin derivative.

Few clinical investigations evaluating the analgesic effectiveness of gabapentin and pregabalin as preventative analgesics for postoperative pain management in patients listed for spine surgery were available in the literature. The preoperative use of gabapentinoids was found to be effective in reducing postoperative pain, total morphine consumption, and morphine-related complications after spine surgery by Liu et al. in their recent meta-analysis of the preoperative use of gabapentinoids for the treatment of acute postoperative pain following spinal surgery. According to their opinion, more research is necessary to ascertain the ideal dosage and whether pregabalin is more effective than gabapentin in managing acute pain following spine surgery [48].

3.6.8 Lignocaine

Lidocaine is a sodium channel blocker and has analgesic, anti-hyperalgesic, and antinociceptive properties. It reduces inputs from injured peripheral nerves and spinal cord neurons and suppresses secondary hyperalgesia by preventing peripheral and central sensitization. Lignocaine has a narrow therapeutic index from 2.5 to 3.5 μg/ml. Intravenous lignocaine given as a 0 to 1.5 mg/kg bolus followed by an infusion of 1.5 to 3 mg/kg/h has improved postoperative pain scores in patients undergoing laparoscopic major abdominal surgery. The effect was observed for 24 h after surgery, with decreased pain scores at rest and on movement. There was an associated decrease in the consumption of postoperative opioids, decreased nausea, and decreased time to first flatus [49]. In a study by Koppert and colleagues, the authors evaluated the preventive analgesic effect of administering intravenous lignocaine 30 min before surgery and continued 24 h postoperatively decreased postoperative pain scores and decreased the amount of morphine consumed overall over the first 72 h following surgery [50]. Use of intravenous lignocaine for pain control has been associated with adverse effects, most notably lightheadedness, dizziness, drowsiness, visual disturbances, metallic taste, or tinnitus. Enhanced recovery after surgery protocols recommend intravenous lignocaine as an opioid-sparing multimodal analgesic adjunct.

3.6.9 Other Drugs

Some other medications and techniques can be used for preventive analgesia, such as tramadol, α-agonist, and intravenous lignocaine. Tramadol is a synthetic opioid that exerts its analgesic effect primarily through a central mechanism and has weak μ-agonist activity. Tramadol also has a peripheral analgesic effect and is used as an adjunct to peripheral blockades. Clonidine is a selective α-agonist that modulates central sensitization and exerts its analgesic effect when administered intrathecally through activation of postsynaptic α-2 receptors in the spinal cord [51]. Bolus dose of Pethidine 10 mg bolus can also be used for PA.

3.6.10 Mechanisms of Preventive Analgesia in Preventing CPSP

The pathophysiology of CPSP involves alterations in the central nervous system, primarily through mechanisms such as central sensitization, which leads to the enhancement of pain perception and the persistence of pain after the resolution of the initial surgical injury. The key mechanism of central sensitization is the increased excitability of neurons in the dorsal horn of the spinal cord and the brain, which results in the amplification of pain signals. Preventive analgesia can help interrupt or modulate this process by controlling nociceptive input during surgery, thus minimizing CNS changes that contribute to the development of CPSP.

3.6.11 Two Essential Conditions for Effective Preventive Analgesia

1. *Effective Suppression of Afferent Input:* To prevent the transition from acute to chronic pain, effective suppression of the afferent pain signals must be achieved. This requires early intervention with analgesic agents that provide sustained pain

relief throughout the perioperative period, especially during the initial postoperative hours when central sensitization is most likely to occur. Key strategies include the use of regional blocks, opioids, NSAIDs, and adjunctive medications such as gabapentinoids or corticosteroids. The duration of analgesia must be adequate to cover the critical time window in which pain sensitization is most likely to occur, typically the first 24–48 h post-surgery.

2. *Combination of Pre-emptive and Maintenance Treatments:* Preventive analgesia extends beyond pre-emptive treatments, such as the administration of analgesics before surgery, to include the maintenance of analgesia throughout the postoperative period. Combining multiple modalities—such as PA, intraoperative pain management, and postoperative therapies—ensures not only that the afferent input is controlled but also that central sensitization is prevented or reversed. In cases where PA does not fully prevent sensitization, additional treatments such as regional blocks or the use of NMDA receptor antagonists (e.g., ketamine) can help in the maintenance of analgesic effects and prevent CPSP.

3.6.12 Preventive Analgesia and CPSP Prevention

The development of CPSP is influenced by various factors, including the type of surgery, the severity of the injury, and the presence of additional risk factors such as preoperative pain, psychological distress, and the use of narcotics during the perioperative period. Effective preventive analgesia aims to manage these risk factors by reducing the magnitude of the injury's nociceptive input, modulating the pain processing pathways, and preventing maladaptive changes in pain perception.

1. *Preemptive Analgesia:* PA, when provided before or at the time of surgery, prevents or reduces the initial nociceptive input that would otherwise lead to sensitization of the

CNS. Common preemptive strategies include the administration of non-opioid analgesics (such as NSAIDs or acetaminophen), regional anesthesia (e.g., epidural analgesia), and the use of gabapentinoids (e.g., pregabalin or gabapentin). This type of intervention aims to modulate the pain pathway before the injury occurs, reducing the likelihood of CPSP.

2. *Maintenance of Analgesia:* Continuation of analgesic therapy in the postoperative period is critical to prevent the development of CPSP. This can involve multimodal analgesia (such as the use of local anesthetics, opioids, and non-steroidal anti-inflammatory drugs) and techniques such as continuous nerve blocks or patient-controlled analgesia (PCA). The objective is to provide sufficient pain relief to prevent the pain-related neuroplasticity that drives central sensitization and subsequent CPSP.
3. *Reversal of Central Sensitization:* In cases where PA is insufficient and central sensitization has already begun, the reversal of these maladaptive changes is key. Strategies include the use of NMDA antagonists (e.g., ketamine), systemic corticosteroids, or α-2 agonists (e.g., clonidine) that modulate central pain processing. These treatments can restore normal pain processing and prevent the transition to chronic pain.

3.6.13 Outcomes and Impact of Preventive Analgesia on CPSP

The evidence supporting preventive analgesia as a strategy to prevent CPSP is compelling. Studies have shown that early and sustained pain control not only improves immediate postoperative recovery but also significantly reduces the incidence of CPSP in high-risk patients. The use of regional anesthesia, for example, has been shown to reduce the incidence of CPSP in major surgeries such as thoracotomies, breast cancer surgeries, and abdominal procedures.

3.7 Conclusion

The concept of preventive analgesia is an essential tool in managing perioperative pain and preventing the long-term development of *CPSP*. By providing effective pain control, modulating nociceptive pathways, and preventing central sensitization, preventive analgesia can significantly reduce the incidence and severity of CPSP, leading to improved patient outcomes and reduced reliance on opioids. Key elements for success include early intervention, multimodal analgesia, and the careful timing of analgesic interventions throughout the perioperative period. A shift towards preventive analgesia and multimodal pain management strategies may offer more reliable outcomes in reducing postoperative pain and improving patient recovery.

References

1. Ji RR, Nackley A, Huh Y, Terrando N, Maixner W. Neuroinflammation and central sensitization in chronic and widespread pain. Anesthesiology. 2018;129(2):343–66.
2. Woolf CJ. Central sensitization: implications for the diagnosis and treatment of pain. Pain. 2011;152(Suppl:3)–S15.
3. Kehlet H, Jensen TS, Woolf CJ. Persistent postsurgical pain: risk factors and prevention. Lancet. 2006;367:1618–25.
4. Kissin I. Preemptive analgesia. Anesthesiology. 2000;93(4):1138–43.
5. Dahl JB, Kehlet H. Preventive analgesia. Curr Opin Anaesthesiol. 2011;24(3):331–8.
6. Møiniche S, Kehlet H, Dahl JB. A qualitative and quantitative systematic review of preemptive analgesia for postoperative pain relief: the role of timing of analgesia. Anesthesiology. 2002;96:725–41.
7. Dahl JB, Kehlet H. The value of pre-emptive analgesia in the treatment of postoperative pain. Br J Anaesth. 1993;70:434–9.
8. Vadivelu N, Mitra S, Schermer E, Kodumudi V, Kaye AD, Urman RD. Preventive analgesia for postoperative pain control: a broader concept. Local Reg Anesth. 2014;7:17–22.
9. Woolf CJ, King AE. Subthreshold components of the cutaneous mechanoreceptive fields of dorsal horn neurons in the rat lumbar spinal cord. J Neurophysiol. 1989;62(4):907–16.
10. Harte SE, Harris RE, Clauw DJ. The neurobiology of central sensitization. J Appl Behav Res. 2018;23:e12137.

11. Simopoulos TT. Chapter 41. Preemptive analgesia. In: Warfield CA, Bajwa ZH, editors. Principles and practice of pain medicine, 2e. The McGraw-Hill Companies; 2004.
12. Latremoliere A, Woolf CJ. Central sensitization: a generator of pain hypersensitivity by central neural plasticity. J Pain. 2009;10:895–926.
13. Dahl JB, Møiniche S. Pre-emptive analgesia. Br Med Bull. 2004;71:13–27.
14. Woolf CJ. Evidence for a central component of post-injury pain hypersensitivity. Nature. 1983;306:686–8.
15. Costigan M, Woolf CJ. Pain: molecular mechanisms. J Pain. 2000;1(Suppl 3):35–44.
16. Lütolf R, Rosner J, Curt A, Hubli M. Indicators of central sensitization in chronic neuropathic pain after spinal cord injury. Eur J Pain. 2022;26(10):2162–75.
17. Butler DS, Moseley GL. Explain Pain. 2nd ed. Adelaide: NOI Group Publications; 2013.
18. Volcheck MM, Graham SM, Fleming KC, Mohabbat AB, Luedtke CA. Central sensitization, chronic pain, and other symptoms: better understanding, better management. Cleve Clin J Med. 2023;90(4):245–54.
19. Doan LV, Blitz J. Preoperative assessment and management of patients with pain and anxiety disorders. Curr Anesthesiol Rep. 2020;10:28–34.
20. Macrae WA, Davies HT. Chronic postsurgical pain. In: Crombie IK, et al., editors. Epidemiology of pain. Seattle: IASP Press; 1999. p. 125–42.
21. Macrae WA. Chronic pain after surgery. Br J Anaesth. 2001;87:88–98.
22. Werner MU, Kongsgaard UE. I. Defining persistent postsurgical pain: is an update required? Br J Anaesth. 2014;113:1–4.
23. Thapa P, Euasobhon P. Chronic postsurgical pain: current evidence for prevention and management. Korean J Pain. 2018;31(3):155–73.
24. Liu SS, Block BM, Wu CL. Effects of perioperative central neuraxial analgesia on outcome after coronary artery bypass surgery: a meta-analysis. Anesthesiology. 2004;101(1):153–61.
25. Ballantyne JC, Carr DB, deFerranti S, Suarez T, Lau J, Chalmers TC, Angelillo IF, Mosteller F. The comparative effects of postoperative analgesic therapies on pulmonary outcome: cumulative meta-analyses of randomized, controlled trials. Anesth Analg. 1998;86(3):598–612.
26. Desai PM. Pain management and pulmonary dysfunction. Crit Care Clin. 1999;15:151–66.
27. Buvanendran A, Kroin JS. Multimodal analgesia for controlling acute postoperative pain. Curr Opin Anaesthesiol. 2009;22:588–93.
28. Wu CL, Fleisher LA. Outcomes research in regional anesthesia and analgesia. Anesth Analg. 2000;91(5):1232–42.
29. Salomaki TE, Laitinen JO, Nuutinen LS. A randomized double-blind comparison of epidural versus intravenous fentanyl infusion for analgesia after thoracotomy. Anesthesiology. 1991;75(5):790–5.

30. Farouk S. Pre-incisional epidural magnesium provides pre-emptive and preventive analgesia in patients undergoing abdominal hysterectomy. Br J Anaesth. 2008;101(5):694–9.
31. Pöpping DM, Elia N, Marret E, Remy C, Tramèr MR. Protective effects of epidural analgesia on pulmonary complications after abdominal and thoracic surgery: a meta-analysis. Arch Surg. 2008;143(10):990–9.
32. Andersen LO, Kehlet H. Analgesic efficacy of local infiltration analgesia in hip and knee arthroplasty: a systematic review. Br J Anaesth. 2014;113(3):360–74.
33. Rosseland LA. No evidence for analgesic effect of intra-articular morphine after knee arthroscopy: a qualitative systematic review. Reg Anesth Pain Med. 2005;30(1):83–93.
34. Svensson CI, Yaksh TL. The spinal phospholipase-cyclooxygenase-prostanoid cascade in nociceptive processing. Annu Rev Pharmacol Toxicol. 2002;42:553–83.
35. Ochroch EA, Mardini IA, Gottschalk A. What is the role of NSAIDs in pre-emptive analgesia? Drugs. 2003;63:2709–23.
36. Li Q, Zhang Z, Cai Z. High-dose ketorolac affects adult spinal fusion: a meta-analysis of the effect of perioperative nonsteroidal anti-inflammatory drugs on spinal fusion. Spine (Phila Pa 1976). 2011;36:7–8.
37. Nussmeier NA, Whelton AA, Brown MT, Langford RM, Hoeft A, Parlow JL, Boyce SW, Verburg KM. Complications of the COX-2 inhibitors parecoxib and valdecoxib after cardiac surgery. N Engl J Med. 2005;352(11):1081–91.
38. Kim YJ, Kim HJ, Kim S, Kim H, Lee CS, Hwang CJ, Cho JH, Ro YJ, Koh WU. Comparison of preemptive and preventive intravenous acetaminophen on opioid consumption in pediatrics undergoing posterior spinal fusion surgery: a randomized controlled trial. Korean J Anesthesiol. 2024;77(3):326–34.
39. Kano K, Kawamura K, Miyake T. Effects of preemptive analgesia with intravenous acetaminophen on postoperative pain relief in patients undergoing third molar surgery: a prospective, single-blind, randomized controlled trial. Med Oral Patol Oral Cir Bucal. 2021;26(1):e64–70.
40. Anderson BJ. Paracetamol (acetaminophen): mechanisms of action. Paediatr Anaesth. 2008;18(10):915–21.
41. Salas S, Frasca M, Planchet-Barraud B, Burucoa B, Pascal M, Lapiana JM, et al. Ketamine analgesic effect by continuous intravenous infusion in refractory cancer pain: considerations about the clinical research in palliative care. J Palliat Med. 2012;15:287–93.
42. Subramaniam K, Subramaniam B, Pawar DK, Kumar L. Evaluation of the safety and efficacy of epidural ketamine combined with morphine for postoperative analgesia after major upper abdominal surgery. J Clin Anesth. 2001;13:339–44.

43. Suski M, Bujak-Gizycka B, Madej J, Kacka K, Dobrogowski J, Woron J, Olszanecki R, Korbut R. Co-administration of dextromethorphan and morphine: reduction of post-operative pain and lack of influence on morphine metabolism. Basic Clin Pharmacol Toxicol. 2010;107(2):680–4.
44. Lavand'homme P. Perioperative pain. Curr Opin Anaesthesiol. 2006;19(5):556–61.
45. Penprase B, Brunetto E, Dahmani E, et al. The efficacy of preemptive analgesia for postoperative pain control: a systematic review of the literature. AORN J. 2015;101(1):94–105.
46. Ben-Menachem E. Pregabalin pharmacology and its relevance to clinical practice. Epilepsia. 2004;45:45–59.
47. Liu B, Liu R, Wang L. A meta-analysis of the preoperative use of gabapentinoids for the treatment of acute postoperative pain following spinal surgery. Medicine (Baltimore). 2017;96(37):e8031.
48. Vigneault L, Turgeon AF, Cote'D, et al. Perioperative intravenous lidocaine infusion for postoperative pain control: a meta-analysis of randomized controlled trials. Can J Anaesth. 2011;58:22–37.
49. Ruscheweyh R, Wilder-Smith O, Drdla R, Liu X-G, Sandkühler J. Long-term potentiation in spinal nociceptive pathways as a novel target for pain therapy. Mol Pain. 2011 Mar 28;7:20.
50. Koppert W, Weigand M, Neumann F, Sittl R, Schuettler J, Schmelz M, Hering W. Perioperative intravenous lidocaine has preventive effects on postoperative pain and morphine consumption after major abdominal surgery. Anesth Analg. 2004;98(4):1050–5.
51. Bahari Z, Meftahi GH. Spinal α_2 -adrenoceptors and neuropathic pain modulation; therapeutic target. Br J Pharmacol. 2019;176(14):2366–81. https://doi.org/10.1111/bph.14580. Epub 2019 Mar 6. PMID: 30657594; PMCID: PMC6592871.

4 Multimodal Approach to Perioperative Analgesia for Commonly Performed Surgeries

Naveen Paliwal and Pooja Bihani

Abstract

Multimodal analgesia is an integrated approach to pain management, combining various pharmacological and non-pharmacological techniques to target different pain pathways. This strategy aims to optimize pain control while reducing opioid use, accelerating recovery, and minimizing side effects. Key principles include the use of non-opioid analgesics, regional analgesia, and non-invasive therapies to provide synergistic effects that enhance pain relief. This chapter delves into the principles and strategies behind the evidence-based multimodal approach to perioperative analgesia, highlighting its benefits in commonly performed procedures and the medications and techniques involved. It emphasizes patient-specific approaches including preemptive analgesia, tailored drug regimens, and continuous nerve blocks for postoperative recovery. By combining multiple techniques, multimodal analgesia not

N. Paliwal
Department of Emergency Medicine, Dr. S.N. Medical College, Jodhpur, India

P. Bihani (✉)
Department of Anaesthesiology, All India Institute of Medical Sciences, Bhubaneswar, Odisha, India

P. Ahluwalia (ed.), *Handbook of Perioperative Analgesia*,
https://doi.org/10.1007/978-981-96-7822-8_4

only enhances the patient's experience but also effectively addresses postoperative morbidity, healthcare costs, and the opioid epidemic.

Keywords

Analgesia · Nerve blocks · Non-opioid analgesics · Opioid epidemic · Pain management · Regional anaesthesia

Key Points

- Multimodal analgesia employs a combination of different classes of medications targeting multiple pain pathways to provide effective pain relief.
- By incorporating non-opioid medications alongside regional anaesthesia, multimodal analgesia significantly reduces opioid requirements, minimizes opioid-related side effects and risks of dependence.
- Preemptive analgesia helps reduce the pain experienced postoperatively by preventing the activation of pain pathways, enhancing overall pain control.
- The multimodal analgesia regimen is individualized based on factors like the type of surgery, patient comorbidities, and pain tolerance, ensuring both effectiveness and safety.

4.1 Introduction

Effective perioperative analgesia is critical in improving patient outcomes, reducing complications, promoting faster recovery, early mobilization, and overall satisfaction. Traditionally, opioid-based analgesia has been the cornerstone of pain management. However, the opioid epidemic has underscored the need for alternative pain management strategies that minimize opioid use [1]. Multimodal analgesia offers a comprehensive approach that reduces opioid use by incorporating a combination of medications and techniques targeting different pain pathways to achieve superior pain control with fewer side effects. By integrating pharmacological agents, regional analgesia, and non-pharmacological interventions, multimodal analgesia enables faster recovery, reduced hospital stays, and lower healthcare costs [2]. The principles of multimodal analgesia, the pharmacology and mechanisms of different analgesic agents, and an evidence-based approach for using multimodal analgesia in common surgical procedures are discussed in this chapter.

4.1.1 Definition and Principles of Multimodal Analgesia

Nociceptive Pain typically arises from tissue injury or inflammation while neuropathic pain results from nerve damage or dysfunction. Perioperative pain arises from the tissue injury and inflammatory response caused by surgical trauma. It involves the activation of nociceptors (pain receptors) in the skin, muscles, and organs. This triggers the release of chemical mediators like prostaglandins, bradykinin, and histamine, which sensitize the nociceptors, leading to pain signals being transmitted to the spinal cord and brain.

The central idea behind multimodal analgesia is to the simultaneous administration of two or more analgesic medications and techniques to target different pain pathways at various levels. By combining various agents, the goal is to achieve superior pain control while minimizing the doses and side effects of each individual drug. Multimodal analgesia can include a combination of non-opioid medications, regional analgesia, and non-pharmacological interventions. It is directed toward four goals: improvement in the patient experience through better pain control, reduction in postoperative morbidity and mortality, reduction in healthcare costs, and decreased physician-contribution to the global opioid epidemic [3].

4.1.2 Key Principles [4]

Synergistic Effect: By using different medications or techniques, multimodal analgesia can produce a synergistic effect, leading to better pain relief.

Reduced Opioid Use: Reducing opioid requirements lowers the risk of opioid-related side effects and enhances patient recovery.

Enhanced Recovery: Better pain control leads to faster mobilization, reduced postoperative complications, and shorter hospital stays.

Patient-Specific Approach: Tailoring the analgesic plan based on patient characteristics, type of surgery, and pain threshold is critical.

4.2 Commonly Used Systemic Analgesic Agents (Table 4.1)

Opioid Analgesics and Opioid Epidemic [13] The opioid discovery has been described as a wonder drug into medical practice for pain management and resulted in an initial surge in opioid usage for perioperative pain management. Most commonly used opioids include morphine, hydromorphone, oxycodone, fentanyl, and its derivatives. Routes of administration varies from oral, intramuscular, transdermal, and intravenous, so it can be utilized in various ways to treat post-surgical pain. Various studies have shown the efficacy of opioids in the perioperative setting to assess their utility in managing acute postoperative pain. Opioids are particularly desirable in setting of quick and rapid rehabilitation, neuropathic pain (buprenorphine and tramadol), acute pain requiring rapid cessation (fentanyl), and others for relieving more visceral experiences of pain (morphine and oxycodone).

Mechanism Opioid medications act by central and peripheral nociception modulator. The opioids that act as agonists at the μ receptor can promote hyperpolarization at both the central and

Table 4.1 Commonly used non-opioid analgesics [5–12]

Medication	Dosage and route of administration	Indication and timing of administration	Side effects/other information
Acetaminophen	PO: 325 mg–1gm every 4–6 h IV: 650 mg–1gm every 4–6 h (maximum-4gm per day)[a]	Mild-to-moderate pain It is often used as a first-line analgesic in the perioperative period	Avoid in severe hepatic disease, acute liver failure Overdose can cause liver injury Not useful in neuropathic pain
NSAIDs and selective COX-2 inhibitor			
Ketorolac	15–30 mg IV every 6–8 h	Mild to moderate pain Preoperative/intra-operative and postoperative period	Abdominal pain GI bleeding Use cautiously in patients taking other anticoagulants Not useful in neuropathic pain Use cautiously in patients with risk of myocardial infarction or stroke especially celecoxib Impaired wound healing
Diclofenac	50-75 mg PO every 6–12 h 75 mg IV every 8–12 h		
Ibuprofen	600–800 mg PO or IV every 6–8 h		
Celecoxib	200–400 mg PO every 12–24 h		
Ketamine	0.25–0.5 mg/kg IV bolus followed by 0.1–0.5 mg/kg/h infusion	Intraoperative pain relief Optimal timing of administration is not defined Postoperative infusion in controlled settings	May result in emergence delirium and hypertension Uncertain optimal dosage regimen Useful adjunct in chronic opioid tolerant patients/cancer pain/chronic persistent postsurgical pain

(continued)

Table 4.1 (continued)

Medication	Dosage and route of administration	Indication and timing of administration	Side effects/other information
Magnesium	30–50 mg/kg IV bolus followed by 6–20 mg/kg/h infusion till the end of surgery or for 4 h after the initial bolus	Preoperative, intraoperative	Uncertain optimal dosage regimen
Dexamethasone	4–8 mg IV every 8 h	Preoperative, intraoperative, and postoperative Adjunct to other analgesic	Also, useful to decrease PONV Transient hyperglycaemia Impaired wound healing
Gabapentinoids			
Gabapentin	300–600 mg PO every 8 h	Preoperative and postoperative period for moderate to severe pain Also useful in neuropathic pain	Synergistic respiratory depression with opioids Dose dependent nausea, vomiting, and dizziness and ataxia Decrease dosage in renal impairment
Pregabalin	75–150 mg every 12 h		
Lignocaine	1 mg/kg bolus followed by 1–2 mg/kg/h infusion	Intraoperative Postoperative in controlled settings	Reduce dosage in liver disease Benefits are shown till 24 h postoperatively
Capsaicin	8% patch; 1–4 patches for 30–60 min every 3 months	Useful for peripheral neuropathic pain	Erythema, Transient hypertension

(continued)

Table 4.1 (continued)

Medication	Dosage and route of administration	Indication and timing of administration	Side effects/other information
Alpha-2 agonist			
Clonidine	1–4 μg/kg IV once 200–300 μg PO once Transdermal patch- 0.2 mg/24 h	Preoperative, intraoperative, and postoperative Useful as adjunct to regional blocks or intra-articular injections	Should monitor for hypotension/bradycardia Considerable opioid sparing effect
Dexmedetomidine	0.5–1 μg/kg IV over 10 min followed by 03–0.7 μg/kg/h infusion		

[a] Weight less than 50 kg or malnutrition, chronic liver disease or chronic alcoholism-maximum dosage 3.75 g/day. *IV* Intravenous, *NSAIDs* non-steroidal anti-inflammatory drugs, *COX-2* Cyclooxygenase-2, *H* hours, *PO* Per oral; *GI* Gastro-intestinal, *PONV* Post-operative nausea and vomiting

peripheral nervous system thereby inhibiting pain signal transmission.

Liberal use of opioid results in significant side effects such as gastric upset, constipation, postoperative nausea and vomiting, respiratory depression, pruritus, and altered mental status or delirium. More concerning is the opioid epidemic which adds to another layer of caution the providers should keep in mind when prescribing opioids, particularly if opioid is used as the only analgesic option for postoperative pain management resulting in more severe the risks of dependence and over usage. In 2017, The Commission on Combating Drug Addiction and the Opioid Crisis report says that approximately 142 Americans were dying every day because of the opioid crisis, and according to the US Center for Disease Control, 130 deaths per day were attributable to the opioid epidemic. The post-surgical pain control with opioid described it a potential contribution to the problem and leading to the creation of chronic opioid addiction in postsurgical patients who were previously opioid naïve which were called the new persistent use of opioid. Therefore, opioids should be used as a reserved or rescue drug as a part of multimodal analgesic regimen. The enhanced recovery after surgery pathways and consensus statement on multimodal analgesia also recommend a standardized protocol of the postoperative pain management with minimal opioid use or opioid free analgesia for better recovery.

4.2.1 Non-opioid Analgesics

Paracetamol (Acetaminophen) [12]*:* A widely used analgesic and antipyretic, paracetamol is effective in managing mild-to-moderate pain and can be administered orally, intravenously, or rectally. According to 2022 multi-society consensus, it is to be used as a first-line analgesic in the perioperative period unless contraindicated due to its safety profile.

Mechanism: Central analgesic effect mediated by activation of descending serotoninergic pathways. It acts by inhibition of prostaglandin synthesis and by its active metabolite i.e. p-aminophenol which act on cannabinoid receptors.

NSAIDs (Non-Steroidal Anti-Inflammatory Drugs) [5]*:* A 2022 multi-society consensus statement recommend routine use of NSAIDs to treat acute perioperative pain in patients without contraindication.

Mechanism: Act by inhibition of cyclooxygenase (COX) enzymes, reducing prostaglandin synthesis, thereby reducing inflammation and pain.

COX-2 Inhibitors (e.g. *Celecoxib*)*:* These selective NSAIDs offer pain relief with a lower risk of gastrointestinal complications. They are useful in surgeries where inflammation contributes to pain but should be used cautiously in patients with cardiovascular issues. Recommendation for routine perioperative use is limited by the overall low quality of data and lack of adverse effects that are clinically significant. Avoid use of celecoxib in patients with sulphonamide toxicity.

Gabapentinoids [6]*:* Originally described as anticonvulsants, gabapentinoids have been extensively used in treatment of chronic neuropathic pain. A meta-analysis on preoperative use of single dose found decrease in postoperative pain and opioid consumption at 24 h. In postoperative period as a part of ERAS protocol, gabapentinoids have been used but optimal dose regimen and timings of administration remain unclear.

Mechanism: Act by depression of dorsal horn sensitivity to pain by multitudes of mechanism. Primarily due to modulation of voltage-gated calcium channels through effect on α2δ-1 subunits, inhibition of descending serotoninergic facilitation, augmentation of descending inhibition, anti-inflammatory action. They also influence the affective component of pain.

Intravenous lignocaine [11]*:* Intravenous (IV) lignocaine has analgesic, anti-inflammatory, and anti-hyperalgesic effects. It is particularly useful in abdominal surgeries, reducing postoperative pain, opioid requirements, and improving bowel recovery. If administered intraoperatively and continued postoperatively in procedures like colorectal surgeries, its use can lead to faster recovery of bowel function and reduced hospital stays. It is mainly effective for controlling visceral pain and improving outcomes in surgeries with high pain potential.

Mechanism: Block sodium channels, preventing nerve impulse propagation.

N-methyl-D-aspartate (NMDA) receptor antagonism (ketamine and magnesium) [8]*:* According to guidelines published by American Society of Regional Anesthesia (ASRA), the subanaesthetic dosage of ketamine infusion should be considered in the patients undergoing surgeries causing severe pain, patients who are opioid dependent or opioid tolerant. Ketamine infusion should be avoided in patients with poorly controlled cardiovascular disease, pregnancy, acute psychosis, severe hepatic dysfunction, elevated intracranial pressure, and elevated intraocular pressure. Primary limiting factor for ketamine use outside operative or intensive care units is its adverse effect such as psychomimetic effects and cardio-vascular effects, so its infusion must be used in the controlled setting under monitoring.

Magnesium sulfate [9]*:* It plays a role in perioperative pain management by modulating pain through the inhibition of N-methyl-D-aspartate (NMDA) receptors, which prevents calcium entry into the cell. This mechanism helps reduce pain perception. Clinical studies have demonstrated that it can decrease postoperative opioid requirements, highlighting its potential for pain control. However, the optimal dosing regimen remains unclear. Systematic reviews have evaluated the effectiveness of magnesium sulfate as a perioperative analgesic in adults undergoing general anaesthesia for abdominal surgeries, comparing its outcomes to those of an inert control.

Mechanism: NMDA receptors antagonist. Can be administered IV or intrathecally. Magnesium has shown a synergism when used in combination to opioid or ketamine.

Alpha-2 Adrenergic Agonists (Dexmedetomidine, Clonidine) [10]*:* They can be used as adjuncts to regional anaesthesia or as systemic analgesics. Dexmedetomidine, in particular, is known for its opioid-sparing properties and is used in surgeries where sedation and pain relief are both required.

Mechanism: These drugs provide analgesia and sedation by acting on alpha-2 adrenergic receptors in the central nervous system.

4.3 Regional Analgesic Techniques in Multimodal Analgesia [14, 15]

Regional analgesia is a cornerstone of multimodal analgesia, providing localized pain control by blocking nerve conduction to the surgical site. This technique significantly reduces the need for systemic opioids and enhances recovery.

Mechanism Regional analgesia involves injection of LA near nerves thereby inhibiting the transmission of nerve signals in sensory, motor, or autonomic nerves. Local anaesthetic is injected near the target nerve, where it disrupts sodium ion channels within the neuronal cell membrane. This prevents the depolarization of nerve cells, blocking the transmission of pain signals (nociceptive signals) from the peripheral nervous system to the central nervous system.

Anaesthesiologists overseeing perioperative pain management should carefully evaluate the risks and benefits for each patient when selecting therapeutic options, which may include neuraxial opioids and local anaesthetics, systemic opioid patient-controlled analgesia (PCA), and peripheral nerve blocks (PNBs). Common forms of regional analgesia are (Table 4.2).

Peripheral Nerve Blocks (PNB) [16, 17]

A PNB is a regional analgesia technique where LA is injected near a specific nerve or group of nerves to block sensation in a particular area of the body. PNB is commonly used for pain management during and after surgical procedures, as well as for diagnostic purposes and chronic pain relief.

Types of PNBs: It can be of single injection block or as continuous nerve block (Catheter Technique) by putting a catheter near the nerve to allow continuous infusion of LA, providing longer-lasting analgesia. Commonly performed PNBs are brachial plexus block (interscalene, supraclavicular, infraclavicular, and axillary blocks, etc.), lower extremity blocks (femoral nerve block, sciatic nerve block), and truncal blocks (intercostal nerve block and paravertebral block). Meta-analysis of randomized controlled trials has reported improved pain relief and reduced analgesic consumption with peripheral nerve blocks.

Advantages of PNBs: Advantages include targeted pain relief, reduced systemic side effects, prolonged postoperative pain relief, reducing the need for opioids and decreased the body's stress response during surgery.

Disadvantages of PNBs include requirement of skill and precision, and improper technique may result in failure or complications. There is risk of nerve injury, potential for temporary or

Table 4.2 Commonly performed regional blocks

Type of block	Area targeted	Common indications	Advantages	Risks
Peripheral nerve block	Specific peripheral nerves (e.g. sciatic, femoral)	Orthopaedic surgeries (e.g. hip, knee, shoulder)	Targeted pain relief, reduces need for general anaesthesia	Nerve injury, local anaesthetic toxicity, incomplete block
Neuraxial block (spinal)	Subarachnoid space (lumbar spine)	Lower abdominal surgeries, lower limb surgeries	Profound motor and sensory blockade, opioid-sparing	Hypotension, spinal headache, infection, nerve damage
Neuraxial block (epidural)	Epidural space (thoracic/ lumbar spine)	Labor analgesia, thoracic/abdominal surgeries	Adjustable blockade, prolonged analgesia, reduced opioids	Hypotension, infection, epidural hematoma, motor blockade
Paravertebral block	Paravertebral space (thoracic/lumbar)	Thoracic surgery, breast surgery, rib fractures	Multi-segmental analgesia, minimal hemodynamic effects	Pneumothorax, infection, local anaesthetic toxicity
Intercostal nerve block	Intercostal nerves (T1-T12)	Rib fractures, thoracotomy, chest trauma	Targeted rib analgesia, simple to perform	Pneumothorax, nerve injury, local anaesthetic toxicity
Fascia Iliaca block	Iliac fascia, femoral and lateral cutaneous nerves	Hip surgery, femur fractures	Safe, easy technique, effective for hip/leg pain	Incomplete block, nerve injury, local anaesthetic toxicity

Transverse abdominis plane (TAP) block	Transversus abdominis plane	Abdominal surgeries (e.g. hernia, C-section)	Effective for lower abdominal pain	Risk of peritoneal injury, incomplete block, local toxicity
PECS block	Pectoral nerves	Breast surgery, thoracic surgery	Opioid-sparing, good chest wall analgesia	Pneumothorax, incomplete block, nerve injury
Rectus sheath block (RSB)	Anterior cutaneous branches of the lower intercostal nerves	Midline abdominal surgeries such as: Umbilical hernia repair Laparoscopic surgeries Incisional hernia repair	Reduces the need for systemic opioids. Simple and easy to perform	Accidental bowel or vascular injury. LAST
Erector Spinae plane block (ESPB)	Dorsal rami of spinal nerves	Thoracic and upper abdominal surgeries: Thoracotomy. Rib fracture. Breast surgery	Provides both visceral and somatic analgesia. Minimal complication due to superficial location	Pneumothorax LAST

(continued)

Table 4.2 (continued)

Quadrates Lumborum block (QLB)	Thoracolumbar fascia and nerves of the lumber plexus (T6 to L1)	Abdominal wall surgeries Hip surgeries Hernia repair Urological surgeries	Visceral and somatic analgesia. Reduce opioid consumption. Longer-lasting pain relief compared to other abdominal wall blocks	Retroperitoneal organ injury. Hematoma
Serratus anterior plane block (SAPB)	Lateral cutaneous branches of the thoracic intercostals nerves	Rib fracture. Mastectomy. Thoracotomy. Chest tube placement.	Minimal hemodynamic changes. Lower risk of pneumothorax	Injury to long thoracic nerve, leading to winged scapula
Interscalene block	Brachial plexus (roots)	Shoulder, upper arm surgery	Effective for shoulder/ upper limb pain	Phrenic nerve block (respiratory compromise), nerve injury
Axillary block	Brachial plexus (terminal branches)	Forearm, hand surgeries	Avoids central complications like phrenic nerve block	Incomplete block, nerve injury, vascular puncture
Popliteal block	Sciatic nerve (popliteal fossa)	Foot and ankle surgeries	Effective foot/ankle analgesia, long-lasting	Nerve injury, local anaesthetic toxicity, hematoma

Femoral nerve block	Femoral nerve (inguinal region)	Hip, knee surgeries, femur fractures	Excellent pain relief for lower limb surgeries	Weakness in quadriceps, nerve injury, local anaesthetic toxicity
Local infiltration	Surgical wound site	Minor surgical procedures, wound closure	Simple, direct pain relief at the surgical site	Infection, local anaesthetic toxicity, short duration
Periarticular injection	Intraarticular space or periarticular tissue	Joint surgeries (e.g. knee, hip, shoulder)	Localized analgesia for joints, easy to perform	Infection, joint damage, short-lasting effect

permanent nerve damage, patchy analgesia leading to discomfort, a risk of infection at the injection or catheter site, a hematoma formation, and transient motor block.

4.3.1 Neuraxial Block Analgesia [18, 19]

Neuraxial block analgesia involves the administration of LA and/or adjuncts into the central nervous system, specifically targeting the spinal cord and nerve roots via the epidural or subarachnoid (intrathecal) spaces. This technique is commonly used to provide analgesia or anaesthesia for surgeries, labour pain, and postoperative pain control.

Types of neuraxial blocks: It can be subarachnoid block (Injection of LA into the subarachnoid space), epidural block (Injection of LA into the epidural space), and combined spinal-epidural (CSE) block.

Advantages of neuraxial block analgesia: Provides superior analgesia compared to systemic opioids, leading to fewer opioid-related side effects, earlier mobilization and shorter hospital stays, especially in major surgeries and target specific block sparing the patient from the global side effects of general anaesthesia, and better hemodynamic stability.

Disadvantages of neuraxial block analgesia: There is risk of hemodymaic disturbances due to physiological sympathetic block following neuraxial block, urinary retention, motor blockade higher concentrations of local anaesthetics, post-dural puncture headache (PDPH), risk of infection and hematoma, neurological complications.

4.3.2 LA Infiltration [20]

Local anaesthetic infiltration involves the injection of a local anaesthetic drug directly into tissues to block pain in a specific area. It is commonly used during minor surgical procedures, dental treatments, and for postoperative pain control. Local anaesthetic infiltration includes intradermal and subcutaneous infiltration, field block, tumescent anaesthesia, and continuous LA infiltration near the surgical site.

Advantages of local anaesthetic infiltration: It provides localized pain control at the site of injection, immediate pain relief for minor procedures, reducing the risk of systemic side effects and early mobilization.

Disadvantages of local anaesthetic infiltration: Disadvantages include a short duration of action, insufficient analgesia, risk of local anesthetic systemic toxicity (LAST), infection and tissue damage.

4.3.3 Periarticular/Intraarticular Injection [21]

Periarticular or intraarticular injections involve administering medication directly into or around a joint space to reduce pain, inflammation, or improve joint function. These injections are commonly used for pain relief in joints affected by arthritis, injuries, or post-surgical conditions. It includes intraarticular injection (drug delivered directly into the joint space) or periarticular injection administered around the joint, targeting the tissues near the joint (ligaments, tendons). Common medications for intraarticular/periarticular injections include local anaesthetics, corticosteroids, hyaluronic acid, platelet rich plasma.

- *Advantages of periarticular/intraarticular injections:* Localized effect, quick pain relief, enhance joint mobility, minimally invasive and long-lasting relief.
- *Disadvantages of periarticular/intraarticular injections:* The effects are often temporary, risk of introducing bacteria into the joint space, leading to septic arthritis, accelerating joint degeneration and inconsistent efficacy.

4.3.4 Truncal Blocks for Analgesia [22, 23]

Truncal blocks are regional anaesthesia techniques that involve injecting LA near the nerves that supply sensation to the trunk of the body, including the chest, abdomen, and lower back. These blocks aim to provide effective analgesia for surgeries or pain in the trunk region by blocking sensory nerve signals from reaching the brain. Types of truncal blocks include transversus abdominis plane block, rectus sheath block, erector spinae plane block, pectoral nerve block, serratus anterior plane block, and quadratus lumborum block.

Advantages: Effective postoperative analgesia, reduced opioid use, selective sensory block, and versatility.

Disadvantages: Limited duration of action, variable success rates, technical expertise, potential complications such as hematoma, infection, or inadvertent injury to nearby structures such as blood vessels or organs.

4.4 Non-invasive Non-pharmacological Therapies [24]

These are complementary and alternative to medical interventions to complement it. These encompass various techniques that may relieve pain through modulation of physiological factors. These techniques can help reduce the reliance on medications, minimize side effects, and enhance patient comfort. Some of the promising options include acupuncture, yoga, tai chi, exercise, and music therapy.

4.4.1 Passively Applied Physical Approaches

Passively applied physical approaches refer to external treatments provided to patients without requiring their active participation. These include complementary and alternative therapies such as acupuncture, massage, transcutaneous electrical nerve stimulation (TENS), and the use of heat or cold packs. Other promising options in this category are practices like yoga, tai chi, exercise, and music therapy.

- *Acupuncture* [25]—Acupuncture is a key component of traditional Chinese medicine that has been used for thousands of years to treat pain. It involves the insertion of thin, sterile needles into specific points on the body, known as acupoints, to stimulate natural healing processes and pain relief. It acts by modulating pain signalling by activation of Aδ and C afferent fibres and release of endorphins. Functional MRI also reveals acupuncture modulates limbic and periaqueductal grey areas involved in affective pain pathway. Evidences also suggests acupuncture may reverse central sensitization also. Safety of acupuncture is good if performed by a trained professional using sterile needles. The risk of complications, such as infection or injury, is very low with mild side effects including soreness, minor bleeding, or bruising at the needle sites.
- *Transcutaneous Electrical Nerve Stimulation (TENS)* [26]*:* It uses electrical stimulation to reduce pain. It acts by activating descending inhibitory pathways and stimulating the production of endogenous pain relievers. Majority of systematic reviews suggest the equivocal effect of TENS due to high risk of bias in the included studies. Used for both acute and chronic pain management.
- *Heat and cold therapy:* Cold therapy reduces blood flow, decreases inflammation, and numbs the area particularly useful in acute injuries. It is applied in the form of ice packs, cold compresses or cooling devices. Heat therapy increases blood flow, relaxes muscles, and alleviates stiffness. It is applied in the form of warm compresses, heating pads, and warm baths.
- *Others:* Ultrasound therapy, electric stimulation, and spinal cord stimulation have also shown to variably affect acute postoperative pain.

4.4.2 Psychological Interventions or Cognitive Behaviour Therapy [27, 28]

Psychological interventions such as cognitive, emotional, or behavioural strategies have been used to modulate pain signals. Mindfulness meditation, guided imagery, avoidance of nocebo effect, deep breathing exercises, humanistic patient centred discussion, sleep hygiene, diet, and social support alter the maladaptive way of patients perceiving and reacting to pain and improves emotional well-being. It acts by increasing endogenous endorphin production and reduction of inflammatory factors.

4.4.3 Distraction [29]

Distraction can have analgesic effects, even additive to placebo treatment. These strategies include music therapy, reading, writing, concentrating on a mental or physical activity, watching movies and therapeutic communication. Not only paediatric patients, but adult and elderly patients also have shown benefit in decreasing acute post-surgical pain as adjunct to pharmacological intervention.

4.5 Others

Preoperative and postoperative education and psychological support, early mobilization, and pre and postoperative physical therapy are essential components of postoperative recovery.

4.6 Preemptive Analgesia [30]

This topic is discussed in detail in chapter on "preemptive analgesia".

4.6.1 The Vital Role of Pre-anaesthesia Check-up to Optimize Perioperative Analgesia Plan [31, 32]

Pre-anaesthesia check-up plays a crucial role in optimizing care for patients with chronic addiction or chronic pain by identifying and addressing specific risks to ensure safe anaesthesia and effective perioperative pain management. It addresses concerns by detailed evaluation of substance use, potential withdrawal symptoms and tolerance issues, pain history and understanding the patient's chronic pain regimen to prevent undermedication or withdrawal. The need for coordination with de-addiction specialists to continue or adjust medication-assist therapies such as methadone or buprenorphine during the perioperative period can be sought. Psychological issues related to addiction and chronic pain, including anxiety and depression, which can complicate perioperative management can be addressed. Lastly, anaesthetic plan is to be tailored in such a way to minimize the risk of relapse, using regional anaesthesia, or non-opioid analgesics when feasible.

Pain assessment tools [33–35]*:* This topic is discussed in detail in chapter on "assessment of pain".

Equipment used: In multimodal analgesia, several types of equipment are employed to administer pain relief and monitor patient safety. Patient-Controlled Analgesia (PCA) Pumps allow patients to self-administer controlled doses of analgesics, typically opioids, to manage their pain effectively. Epidural Infusion Pumps are used to deliver continuous or intermittent doses of LA and opioids through an epidural catheter for effective pain control, especially postoperatively. PNB Catheters, combined with infusion pumps, provide targeted pain relief by delivering LA near specific nerves, minimizing the need for systemic opioids. Nerve blocks should ideally be administered under direct visualization using ultrasound to precisely guide the delivery of LA around targeted nerves. This technique enhances the safety and effectiveness of regional anaesthesia. The recommended dosing regimen of commonly used local anaesthetic is summarized in Table 4.3.

Documentation of Perioperative Analgesia Perioperative analgesia documentation is crucial for patient safety, legal accountability, and effective pain management. It should include a thorough preoperative pain assessment, noting patient history, risk factors, and consent. During surgery, all analgesic medications, dosages, and routes must be recorded, along with intraoperative monitoring and any complications. Postoperative documentation includes regular pain assessments, details of medications and non-pharmacological interventions, management of side effects, and patient education. Finally, discharge instructions, including pain control measures and follow-up plans, should be clearly documented, ensuring comprehensive care throughout the perioperative period.

Table 4.3 Recommended dosing regimen of commonly used local anaesthetic for regional analgesia

Analgesic regimen	Bupivacaine	Levobupivacaine	Ropivacaine
Patient controlled epidural analgesia	0.05%–0.1% solution @ 4-6 ml/h Demand dose: 2–4 ml Lockout interval: 10-15 min	0.05%–0.1% solution @ 4–6 ml/h Demand dose: 2–4 ml Lockout interval: 10-15 min	0.1%–0.2% solution @ 3–5 ml/h Demand dose: 2–5 ml Lockout time: 20 min
Peripheral nerve block (single shot)	0.125%–0.5% (150 mg)	0.125%–0.5% (150 mg)	0.2%–0.5% (200 mg)
Peripheral nerve block (continuous infusion)	4-15 ml/h of 0.1%–0.125% solution (not to exceed 2 mg/kg over 4 h or maximum total dose of 400 mg in 24 h)	4-15 ml/h of 0.1%–0.125% solution (not to exceed 2 mg/kg over 4 hours or maximum total dose of 400 mg in 24 h)	5-10 ml/hour of 0.2% solution (not to exceed 3 mg/kg in 4 h or maximum total dose of 800 mg in 24 h)

A Prototype Perioperative Analgesia Documentation Proforma

1. Patient Information:
   - Name: ________Age/Gender: _________Medical Record Number: __________________.
2. Preoperative assessment and analgesia plan.
   - Pain history________________.
   - Baseline Pain Score (0–10): ____Risk Factors: Opioid Use/Tolerance: __ Yes __ No.
   - Allergies/Adverse Drug Reactions:____________________.
   - Patient Consent Obtained for Analgesia Plan: __ Yes __ No.
   - Preoperative Analgesia Plan:

     Medications: ________Dose ______Time____.

     Non-pharmacological Methods: ________.

     Block/regional analgesia plan.

     Patient counselling.
3. Intraoperative pain control strategies: (Tick all that apply).
   - General Anaesthesia/ regional anaesthesia/ combined.
   - Medications Administered:

Medication	Dose	Route	Time Given
______________	__________	_________	___________

4. Postoperative Analgesia:
   - Pain Assessments (Specify time intervals):

Time	Pain Score (0–10)	Additional Comments
_______	_________________	___________________

   - Medications Administered Postoperatively:

Medication	Dose	Route	Time Given
______________	__________	_________	___________

   - Non-pharmacological Interventions:
   - Rescue opioid analgesic:

- Adverse events, if any: ____________________.
- Management of Side Effects: ______________________.

5. Discharge and Follow-up advice:
   - Pain Score at Discharge: _______________.
   - Discharge Analgesia Plan:

Medication	Dose	Frequency	Duration
____________	_________	_________	_______

   - Patient Education Provided: Yes/No.
   - Follow-up advice: ______________________________.
6. Additional Notes:

   Signature of Anesthesiologist.

   Date: ______________________.

Future Trends in Perioperative Analgesia Artificial Intelligence (AI) is transforming pain assessment by providing objective, accurate, and personalized insights, overcoming the limitations of traditional self-reporting methods. Machine learning and AI can analyze self-report measures, physiological data such as facial expressions, voice patterns, and biometrics and/or medical records, to create algorithms to better assess pain non-invasively. It potentially enables personalized pain management by predicting the most effective treatments based on individual patient data and history and supports remote monitoring through AI-enabled devices and apps, ensuring timely interventions. AI also aids in predictive analytics, identifying patients at risk for chronic pain or complications, and offers enhanced decision support for clinicians, leading to more precise and holistic pain management strategies.

Every health care institution must prepare their own protocols and come up with analgesic regimens for providing effective pain relief for various surgical procedures. These should be prepared based upon available literature and scientific evidence and must be revised on time to time basis. One such example of providing analgesia in patients undergoing total hip replacement is discussed below.

4.7 Principles of Multimodal Analgesia for Total Hip Arthroplasty [36–38]

Hip orthopaedic surgeries, such as total hip arthroplasty (THA), hip fracture repair, and hip resurfacing, can lead to significant postoperative pain, making effective analgesia critical for enhanced recovery and rehabilitation. Multimodal analgesia is essential in these surgeries as it aims to control pain through a combination of medications and techniques, thereby improving outcomes and reducing opioid use. (Table 4.4).

Table 4.4 Evidence-based recommendation for total hip arthroplasty [38]

Timing of intervention	Recommended interventions	Interventions that lack or insufficient evidences
Pre-operative	Prehabilitation and education Consider giving paracetamol + NSAID/COX-2 inhibitors on the morning of surgery as preemptive analgesia	Carbohydrate preloading
Intra-operative	General/spinal anaesthesia (if spinal block for surgery, consider adding intrathecal morphine 0.1 mg) Paracetamol + NSAID/COX-2 inhibitors + Dexamethasone 8–10 mg IV + Consider performing peripheral nerve block as per the recommendations	Gabapentinoids Ketamine Lateral femoral cutaneous block Anterior quadrates lumborum block Femoral nerve block Lumbar plexus block Epidural analgesia Local infiltration adjuncts to local anaesthesia drugs or local infiltration infusion or repeated injections Pericapsular infiltration of local anaesthetic
Postoperative interventions	Paracetamol + NSAID/COX-2 inhibitors Opioids for rescue Consider prescribing PCA using opioid medications OR LA infiltration through perineural catheter if placed	Tranexamic acid Partial weight bearing Topical fibrin sealant TENS

4.8 Conclusion

Multimodal analgesia represents a paradigm shift in postoperative pain management. By leveraging a combination of analgesic agents and regional techniques, this approach minimizes opioid consumption, enhances recovery, and improves patient outcomes. Tailoring analgesic protocols to individual patient needs and utilizing preemptive analgesia further optimizes pain control while reducing complications. As healthcare moves toward opioid-sparing strategies, multimodal analgesia stands as an essential component of enhanced recovery pathways, offering a holistic and patient-centred approach to perioperative pain management.

References

1. Alexander GC, Kruszewski SP, Webster DW. Rethinking opioid prescribing to protect patient safety and public health. JAMA. 2012;308(18):1865–6.
2. Schwenk ES, Mariano ER. Designing the ideal perioperative pain management plan starts with multimodal analgesia. Korean J Anesthesiol. 2018;71:345–52.
3. Chou R, Gordon DB, de Leon-Casasola OA, Rosenberg JM, Bickler S, Brennan T, et al. Management of postoperative pain: a clinical practice guideline from the American Pain Society, the American Society of Regional Anesthesia and Pain Medicine, and the American Society of Anesthesiologists' Committee on Regional Anesthesia, Executive Committee, and Administrative Council. J Pain. 2016;17:131–57.
4. Mariano ER, Dickerson DM, Szokol JW, Harned M, Mueller JT, Philip BK, et al. A multisociety organizational consensus process to define guiding principles for acute perioperative pain management. Reg Anesth Pain Med. 2022;47:118–27.
5. Ramaswamy S, Wilson JA, Colvin L. Non-opioid-based adjuvant analgesia in perioperative care. Continuing Education in Anaesthesia, Critical Care and Pain. 2013;13(5):152–7.
6. Davari M, Amani B, Amani B, Khanijahani A, Akbarzadeh A, Shabestan R. Pregabalin and gabapentin in neuropathic pain management after spinal cord injury: a systematic review and meta-analysis. Korean J Pain. 2020;33:3–12.
7. Guy S, Mehta S, Leff L, Teasell R, Loh E. Anticonvulsant medication use for the management of pain following spinal cord injury: systematic review and effectiveness analysis. Spinal Cord. 2014;52:89–96.

8. Schwenk ES, Viscusi ER, Buvanendran A, Hurley RW, Wasan AD, Narouze S, et al. Consensus guidelines on the use of intravenous ketamine infusions for acute pain management from the American society of Regional Anesthesia and Pain Medicine, the American Academy of Pain Medicine, and the American Society of Anesthesiologists. Reg Anesth Pain Med. 2018;43:456–66.
9. Avci Y, Rajarathinam M, Kalsekar N, Tawfic Q, Krause S, Nguyen D, et al. Unravelling the analgesic effects of perioperative magnesium in general abdominal surgery: a systematic review and meta-analysis of randomized controlled trials. Braz J Anesthesiol. 2024;74:844524.
10. Giovannitti JA Jr, Thoms SM, Crawford JJ. Alpha-2 adrenergic receptor agonists: a review of current clinical applications. Anesth Prog. 2015;62(Spring):31–9.
11. Foo I, Macfarlane AJ, Srivastava D, et al. The use of intravenous lignocaine for postoperative pain and recovery: international consensus statement on efficacy and safety. Anaesthesia. 2021;76:238–50.
12. Freo U, Ruocco C, Valerio A, Scagnol I, Nisoli E. Paracetamol: a review of guideline recommendations. J Clin Med. 2021;10:3420.
13. Nicholas TA 4th, Robinson R. Multimodal analgesia in the era of the opioid epidemic. Surg Clin North Am. 2022;102:105–15.
14. Chen YK, Boden KA, Schreiber KL. The role of regional anaesthesia and multimodal analgesia in the prevention of chronic postoperative pain: a narrative review. Anaesthesia. 2021;76:8–17.
15. O'Neill A, Lirk P. Multimodal analgesia. Anesthesiol Clin. 2022;40:455–68.
16. Ní Eochagáin A, Carolan S, Buggy DJ. Regional anaesthesia truncal blocks for acute postoperative pain and recovery: a narrative review. Br J Anaesth. 2024;132:1133–45.
17. El-Boghdadly K, Levy NA, Fawcett WJ, Knaggs RD, Laycock H, Baird E, et al. Peri-operative pain management in adults: a multidisciplinary consensus statement from the Association of Anaesthetists and the British Pain Society. Anaesthesia. 2024;79:1220. https://doi.org/10.1111/anae.16391.
18. Leander M, Loon V, Lopez K, Ana M. Role of regional anesthesia in Enhanced Recovery After Surgery (ERAS) protocols. Curr Opin Anaesthesiol. 2021;34:616–25.
19. Memtsoudis SG, Poeran J, Zubizarreta N, Cozowicz C, Mörwald EE, Edward R. Association of multimodal pain management strategies with perioperative outcomes and resource utilization: a population-based study. Anesthesiology. 2018;128:891–902.
20. Li X, Yu L, Yang J, Tan H. Multimodal analgesia with ropivacaine wound infiltration and intravenous flurbiprofen axetil provides enhanced analgesic effects after radical thyroidectomy: a randomized controlled trial. BMC Anesthesiol. 2019;19:167.

21. Chandrashekaraiah MM, Shah VH, Sahitya PV, Pandey VC, Butt AJ, Mohammed S, et al. Impact of intra-articular local anesthesia infiltration versus femoral nerve block for postoperative pain management in total knee arthroplasty. Anesth Essays Res. 2021;15:208–12.
22. Arunangshu C, Rakhi K, Datta T. Ultrasound-guided truncal blocks: a new frontier in regional anaesthesia. Indian J Anaesth. 2016;60:703–11.
23. Paliwal N, Maurya N, Suthar OP, Janweja S. Segmental thoracic spinal anesthesia versus general anesthesia for breast cancer surgery: a prospective randomized-controlled open-label trial. J Anaesthesiol Clin Pharmacol. 2022;38:560–5.
24. Shi Y, Wu W. Multimodal non-invasive non-pharmacological therapies for chronic pain: mechanisms and progress. BMC Med. 2023;21:372.
25. Nielsen A, Dusek JA, Taylor-Swanson L, Tick H. Acupuncture therapy as an evidence-based nonpharmacologic strategy for comprehensive acute pain care: the academic consortium pain task force white paper update. Pain Med. 2022;23:1582–612.
26. Vance CGT, Dailey DL, Chimenti RL, Van Gorp BJ, Crofford LJ, Sluka KA. Using TENS for pain control: update on the state of the evidence. Medicina. 2022;58:1332.
27. Lim JA, Choi SH, Lee WJ, Jang JH, Moon JY, Kim YC, et al. Cognitive-behavioral therapy for patients with chronic pain: implications of gender differences in empathy. Medicine (Baltimore). 2018;97:e10867.
28. Arrow K, Burgoyne LL, Cyna AM. Implications of nocebo in anaestheisa care. Anaesthesia. 2022;77:11–20.
29. Miller K, Rodger S, Bucolo S, Greer R, Kimble RM, Multi-modal Distraction. Using technology to combat pain in young children with burn injuries. Burns. 2010;36:647–58.
30. Rosero EB, Joshi GP. Preemptive, preventive, multimodal analgesia: what do they really mean? Plast Reconstr Surg. 2014;134:85S–93S.
31. Jaju R, Varshney S, Bihani P, Paliwal N, Karim HMR, Bhuyan D. Enhanced perioperative communication elevates patients' understanding, perception, and satisfaction for anesthesia services: insights from a survey study. Saudi J Anesth. 2024;18:376–87.
32. Kaye AD, Kandregula S, Kosty J, Sin A, Guthikonda B, Ghali GE, et al. Chronic pain and substance abuse disorders: preoperative assessment and optimization strategies. Best Pract Res Clin Anaesthesiol. 2020;34:255–67.
33. Dydyk AM, Grandhe S. Pain Assessment. In: StatPearls [internet]. Treasure Island. FL: StatPearls Publishing; 2024 Jan.
34. El-Tallawy SN, Pergolizzi JV, Vasiliu-Feltes I, Ahmed RS, LeQuang JK, El-Tallawy HN, et al. Incorporation of "artificial intelligence" for objective pain assessment: a comprehensive review. Pain Ther. 2024;13:293–317.

35. Bihani P, Pandey A, Jha M, Paliwal N, Jaju R, Solanki RK. Comparing perfusion index and visual analogue scores for postoperative pain assessment following upper limb surgeries under supraclavicular brachial plexus block: an observational study. Cureus. 2024;16(3):e55529.
36. Hadzic A. Textbook of regional anesthesia and acute pain management. McGraw Hill; 2017.
37. Chunduri A, Aggarwal AK. Multimodal pain management in orthopedic surgery. J Clin Med. 2022;11:6386.
38. Anger M, Valovska T, Beloeil H, Lirk P, Joshi GP, Van de Velde M, et al. PROSPECT Working Group* and the European Society of Regional Anaesthesia and Pain Therapy. PROSPECT guideline for total hip arthroplasty: a systematic review and procedure-specific postoperative pain management recommendations. Anaesthesia. 2021;76:1082–97.

Drugs for Acute Pain Management

5

Damarla Haritha and Soumya Sarkar

Abstract

Pain, an unpleasant sensory and emotional experience due to actual or potential tissue damage, is subjective and influenced by multiple factors, which makes management challenging. The majority of patients experience moderate to severe pain after surgery, and inadequate pain management often leads to delirium, delayed recovery, and chronic pain. Effective pain management requires a spectrum of multimodal approaches, including systemic pharmacological therapies, local infiltration techniques, neuraxial & regional analgesia, and non-pharmacological methods like acupuncture or transcutaneous electrical nerve stimulation (TENS). Multimodal regimens combining different classes are often recommended to maximize efficacy and reduce the risks of opioid use and other adverse effects. However, each modality operates through different mechanisms along the pain pathway. This chapter

D. Haritha
Department of Anesthesiology, Narayana Medical College, Nellore, India

S. Sarkar (✉)
Department of Anesthesiology, All India Institute of Medical Sciences (AIIMS), Kalyani, Kalyani, India

P. Ahluwalia (ed.), *Handbook of Perioperative Analgesia*,
https://doi.org/10.1007/978-981-96-7822-8_5

addresses the different modalities' distinct uses, side effects, and potential complications.

Keywords

Perioperative pain management · Multimodal analgesia · Opioid and non-opioid analgesics

Key Points
- Definition and challenges of perioperative pain management
- Classification of pain
- Impact of inadequate pain management
- WHO pain ladder
- Multimodal management strategies

5.1 Introduction

Pain is defined as 'the unpleasant sensory and emotional experience associated with or resembling that associated with actual or potential tissue damage' as per the International Association for the Study of Pain in 2020 [1]. The subjective nature of pain and the influence of various socio-cultural factors on the perception make management of acute pain in the postoperative setting highly challenging [2]. Current literature suggests that approximately 80% of the patients experience moderate to severe pain in the perioperative period, which might even be higher in low-resource countries [3]. Inadequately managed pain in the immediate postoperative period had been associated with an elevated risk of complications such as delirium, delayed ambulation and discharge, increased morbidity, poor perioperative outcomes, and worst of all development of chronic pain [4–8]. Acute pain after surgery can be classified as nociceptive (mediated by unmyelinated C fibres, thinly myelinated Ad fibres and myelinated Ab fibres), inflammatory (mediated by cytokines in response to tissue inflammation), or neuropathic (due to increased axonal sensitivity following neural injury) [2]. Also, it is classified as somatic (originating in the cutaneous and deep tissues), which is more sharp and localized, and visceral (originating from the visceral organs), which is a dull, aching, and more generalized type of pain [9].

The easiest way to understand pain management is the WHO step ladder approach, initially introduced in 1986 for treating cancer pain. Over the years, many modifications have been suggested, and their use has been extended to other acute and chronic pain types. The original ladder had three steps, but the most recent revision included the addition of a fourth step and also stressed the bi-directional manner one can approach [10]. The original intention was to start the patient on the mildest analgesics and escalate as and when required. However, the most potent analgesic can be used for the shortest duration possible and quickly tapered off in acute pain (Fig. 5.1).

The various modalities to treat pain post-surgery include:

1. Systemic pharmacological therapy
2. Topical, local infiltration techniques
3. Neuraxial analgesia
4. Regional anaesthetic procedures
5. Non-pharmacological therapies such as acupuncture, acupressure, hypnosis, and transcutaneous electrical nerve stimulation (TENS)

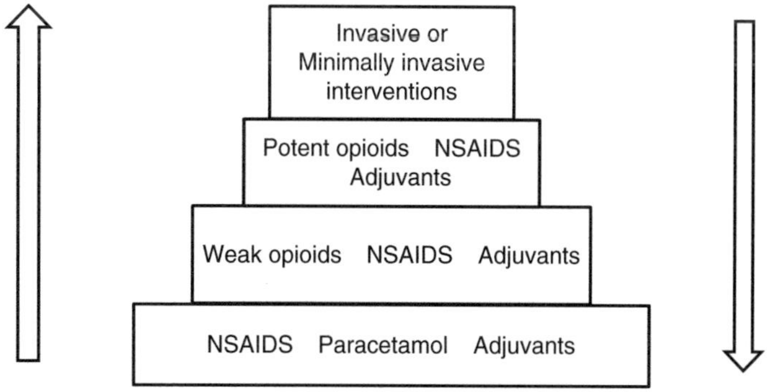

Fig. 5.1 WHO step ladder for pain management

Below is a brief overview of the pharmacological agents used to treat acute pain after surgery.

5.2 Pharmacological Agents

The simplest way to classify the pharmacological agents is based on their mechanism of action along the pain pathway and how they act to relieve or stop the pain (Fig. 5.2). A brief discussion about each drug group's classification, mechanism of action, uses, and various complications are as follows.

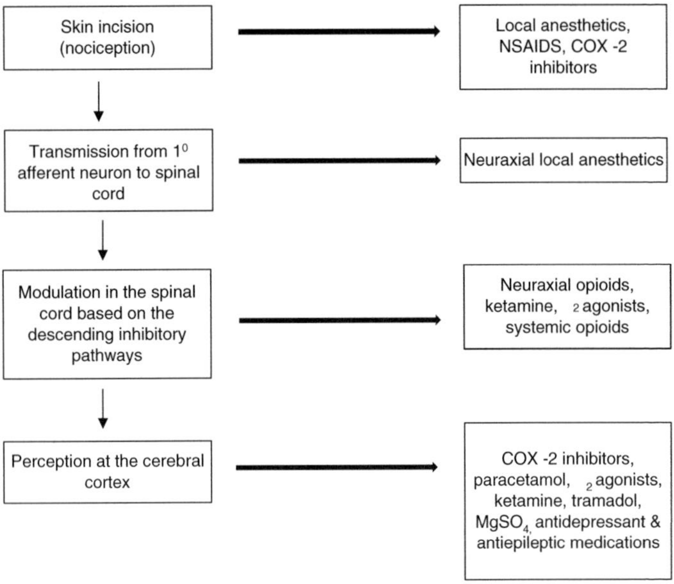

Fig. 5.2 Pain pathway and site of action of various drugs

5.3 Local Anaesthetics

All the local anaesthetics include a lipophilic amine and a hydrophilic ester group, joined together by an intermediate link. Based on the nature of this link, local anaesthetics are roughly divided into esters (e.g. cocaine, chloroprocaine) and amides (e.g. lignocaine, bupivacaine, levobupivacaine and ropivacaine). The primary mechanism of action is suppression of the formation of action potential by inhibiting the voltage-gated Na + channels at the nerve terminals, preventing the nociception [11].Lignocaine is also postulated to have anti-inflammatory, anti-metastatic, and antibacterial properties. Route of administration includes topical (EMLA (Eutectic mixture of Local Anaesthetics) to skin, 10% lignocaine spray for mucosa, lignocaine gel), subcutaneous, intravenous (lignocaine for systemic analgesia, prilocaine for intravenous regional anaesthesia), perineural (for regional blocks), epidural, and intrathecal. Notable side effects are allergic reactions, local toxicity causing tissue necrosis, methemoglobinemia with prilocaine, transient neurological symptoms, and sedation with lignocaine [12].

The most dreaded complication includes Local Anesthetic Systemic Toxicity (LAST). The reported incidence is highly variable in the literature, ranging from 25 per 10,000 nerve blockades to nil in 12,000 nerve blocks [13]. Accidental intravascular injection is the most common cause but can also occur when one exceeds the recommended maximum dose. The two main organs affected are the heart and brain. Neurological CNS manifestations such as seizures, confusion, hallucination, perioral tingling, and numbness are noted, and cardiovascular CVS symptoms include arrhythmias, hypotension, ST—T changes, dyspnea, chest pain, cardiac arrest, etc. Bupivacaine, the most lipophilic of the local anaesthetics with a longer duration of action, has predominant cardiac symptoms when the intravascular spread is noted. Diagnosis is often clinical, based on a high index of suspicion and relevant history. Initial management is mainly focused on standard A (airway), B (breathing), and C (circulation). Benzodiazepines are used for the treatment of seizures. The mainstay of therapy is an intravenous 100 ml bolus of 20% intralipid emulsion (1.5 ml/kg over 2–3 min) followed by 250 ml infusion (0.25 ml/kg/min) over 20–30 min [14]. The bolus can be repeated three times maximum and infusion dose doubled if there is no improvement in hemodynamics [14]. Beta blockers, calcium channel blockers, and vasopressin are avoided during resuscitation and lower doses of epinephrine than standard 1 mg are recommended in case of cardiac arrest [14]. Once the patient is stable, it is advisable to monitor at least 2 h after the last seizure, 4–6 h after the cardiovascular instability and as long as appropriate after cardiac arrest [14]. Newer formulations such as liposomal bupivacaine and SABER (Sucrose acetate isobutyrate extended release) bupivacaine allow a longer duration of action, reducing the cumulative dose requirement [14]. The American Society of Anesthesiologists (ASA) committee on regional anaesthesia recommends regular usage of surgical site-specific topical, infiltration, or regional anaesthetic techniques in all surgeries and also the use of neuraxial techniques in all major abdominal and thoracic procedures in patients with high-risk complications [15].

Intravenous agents can be discussed briefly as:

1. Opioids
2. Non-opioid analgesics

5.3.1 Opioids

Opioids form the mainstay of treatment for postoperative pain. The first opioid, morphine, was discovered in 1806 from opium poppy *Papaver Somniferum,* giving all its derivatives the name ‘opioids’ [16]. They can be broadly classified as natural (morphine, codeine, thebaine, and papaverine), semi-synthetic (heroin, buprenorphine, hydromorphone), and synthetic (fentanyl, pethidine, methadone), etc. The opioid receptors are present throughout the central nervous system (CNS), gastrointestinal tract (GIT), heart, vas deferens, etc., and are of three types: mu (μ), kappa (k), delta (δ) and non-classical receptors like nociceptin, orphanin [17]. Based on the action at the receptors, they are further classified as agonists (morphine, fentanyl), antagonists (naloxone), and partial agonist–antagonists (nalbuphine, buprenorphine).

Even though they have been the oldest analgesics available, their usage has become questionable due to their tendency for addiction, tolerance, and various side effects. Opioids are used for severe, chronic, and cancer pain and should not be prescribed for longer duration. The routes of administration depend on the drug and include oral, topical, transdermal patches, intramuscular, intravenous, and neuraxial. ASA recommends the usage of oral over systemic administration and intravenous patient-controlled analgesia (PCA) rather than continuous infusion if systemic use is deemed necessary [15]. Adverse effects include sedation, pruritis, urinary retention, respiratory depression, hypotension, histamine release, constipation, nausea and vomiting, postoperative ileus, and tolerance, sometimes leading to hyperalgesia. All the patients who receive opioids in the perioperative period should be monitored for these conditions based on the duration of action of the drug administered. Respiratory depression is the most dreaded complication due to the activation of opioid receptors in the respiratory centre of the brain stem, leading to hypoventilation and carbon dioxide retention [18]. Clinical symptoms include altered mentation, reduced respiratory rate, and pinpoint pupils, described as the classical triad of opioid overdose [19]. Naloxone, a competitive antagonist of opioid receptors, is the drug of choice apart from supportive management. An initial bolus of 0.1 mg/kg is administered intravenously, and the duration of action is approximately 30–45 min. An infusion should follow it in case toxicity of long-acting opioids is suspected [18].

5.3.1.1 Tramadol

Even though tramadol is structurally related to morphine and codeine, it is generally not categorized as a typical opioid compound. It is the only non-scheduled opioid as per the FDA and is widely used for the treatment of mild to moderate pain on an over-the-counter basis around the world [20]. It has dual analgesic action as a m receptor agonist and prevents serotonin and norepinephrine reuptake. It is available in oral, per rectal, and parenteral formulations. The recommended maximum dose is 400 mg per day and 300 mg per day for extended-release preparations [20]. Metabolism is via CYP 450 mediated phase I reaction in the liver followed by conjugation in phase II reaction. Active metabolites include O -desmethyl tramadol and N, O—desmethyl tramadol, which can accumulate in patients with renal dysfunction, leading to prolonged duration of action.

It is generally preferred in patients in whom cardiorespiratory compromise must be avoided, such as obstructive sleep apnoea, hypoventilation syndromes, chronic obstructive pulmonary disease, and elderly patients for perioperative analgesia. Another routine use of tramadol is for the treatment of postoperative shivering. It is also postulated to prevent catheter-related bladder discomfort and voiding urgency [21]. Side effects include dizziness, nausea, vomiting, sweating, dry mouth, and diarrhoea. Rarely, there can be allergic reactions and cardiovascular compromise like arrhythmias, hypotension, and shock.

5.3.1.2 Tapentadol

It is a centrally acting analgesic, acts as a μ-opioid receptor agonist and, inhibits the reuptake of norepinephrine, enhances descending inhibitory pain pathways, reduces pain perception. It is effective for both nociceptive and neuropathic pain. Tapentadol provides analgesia with fewer side effects compared to pure opioids like morphine due to its dual mode of action. Depending on pain severity, the recommended dose is 50–100 mg every 4–6 h [22]. The maximum dose is 600 mg daily for short-term acute pain management. It can potentiate the sedative effects of alcohol, benzodiazepines, and other central nervous system depressants. Concurrent use with monoamine oxidase inhibitors (MAOIs) can lead to serotonin syndrome or hypertensive crisis. It has similar efficacy to higher-dose opioids for acute pain with fewer gastrointestinal side effects. Thus, it can be a potential first-line opioid of choice for acute pain management, balancing adequate analgesia with a lower risk of adverse gastrointestinal events [22].

5.3.2 Non-opioid Analgesics

5.3.2.1 Non-steroidal Anti-inflammatory Drugs

NSAIDs are anti-inflammatory, antipyretic, antiplatelet, and analgesic agents that inhibit cyclo-oxygenase (COX) enzyme, limiting prostaglandin production and affecting nociception. They are widely used for the treatment of mild to moderate pain in the perioperative setting due to their proven opioid-sparing effect [23]. Brief classification based on the chemical structure is described in Table 5.1. Based on the selectivity of the COX inhibition, they are divided into nonselective (e.g. aspirin, diclofenac, ibuprofen, etc.) and selective COX—2 inhibitors (e.g. celecoxib, etoricoxib) [24].

The various routes of administration include topical, oral, rectal, intramuscular, and intravenous administration based on the drug and available formulations. Dosage also depends on the individual drugs, but the lowest possible dosage is recommended for the shortest duration. The common side effects include hypersensitivity reactions, nephrotoxicity, gastric ulceration, thromboembolic events, reduced seizure threshold, and hepatotoxicity [25]. Contraindications include active bleeding, peptic ulcer disease, uncontrolled hypertension, elderly age, coronary bypass grafting, stroke, and myocardial infarction (excluding aspirin). COX-2 inhibitors have improved gastric safety profiles, but removing rofecoxib from the market due to its adverse cardiovascular effect suggests their use needs to be more strategic [26]. The ASA recommendations also suggest routine usage of NSAIDs such as paracetamol as part of the multimodal regimen of analgesia unless contraindicated [15].

Table 5.1 Classification of non-steroidal anti-inflammatory drugs (NSAIDs)

Chemical structure	Examples
Acetylated salicylates	Aspirin
Acetic acid derivatives	Diclofenac, indomethacin
Propionic acid derivatives	Naproxen, ibuprofen
Anthranilic acid derivatives	Piroxicam, meloxicam
Enolic acids	Mefenamic acid

5.3.2.2 Paracetamol

Paracetamol is the most commonly used antipyretic analgesic medication used around the world and is available on an over-the-counter basis. Even though pharmacodynamics resembles that of NSAIDS, the mechanism of action of this drug remains unknown. It doesn't bind to either COX −1 or COX −2. Still, it is believed to antagonize the COX −3 enzyme, which results in decreased prostaglandin synthesis in the central nervous system, causing analgesia via the serotonergic pathway and antipyresis via the hypothalamic heat-regulating centre [25]. It is routinely used in mild to moderate pain and for reduction of temperature in fever.

It had been shown to have equianalgesic efficacy to appropriate doses of NSAIDS, tramadol and 10 mg morphine, but with reduced side effects [27]. Paracetamol is not adequate for neuropathic pain but provides good analgesia in musculoskeletal pain. It is found to have an opioid-sparing impact as part of a multimodal regimen. It is also proven to act synergistically with other drugs such as NSAIDS, tramadol, codeine, caffeine, etc. [27]. It is administered via intravenous, intramuscular, oral, per rectal route, and there was no significant difference in pain scores between patients who were given intravenous and oral formulation one hour after administration in dental extraction [27].

Oral bioavailability is between 63% and 89% in adults [28]. It is mainly metabolized in the liver through glucuronidation and sulphation into non-toxic metabolites. Still, a small amount (5–10%) undergoes oxidation to form N-acetyl-p-benzoquinone imine (NAPQI), which is highly toxic and is responsible for acute hepatic necrosis in paracetamol overdose [27]. NAPQI is detoxified by conjugation and glucuronidation in the liver to mercapturic acid and excreted through the kidney. But when paracetamol is administered in higher doses, sulphation becomes saturated, and a larger amount (10%) of the drug gets metabolized to NAPQI, reducing the glutathione reserves of the liver and causing cell death. The maximum recommended dose for an adult with creatinine clearance >30 ml/min is 4 gm daily [27]. In children <10 kg, 7.5 mg/kg and >10 kg, 15 mg/kg dosing is recommended [27].

Side effects are rare and generally well tolerated in all age groups. Commonly encountered side effects include allergic reactions, Steven Johnson syndrome, pancytopenia, electrolyte abnormalities, etc. The most life-threatening complication is acute hepatic failure due to paracetamol poisoning. Initial management is generally supportive, and N—Acetylcysteine (NAC) is the drug of choice for definitive treatment [28]. NAC helps in the restoration of the glutathione pool, which is depleted by NAPQI and prevents further cell injury.

5.3.2.3 Ketamine

Ketamine is a phencyclidine derivative which was routinely used as an induction agent, sedative and premedication. Its potent analgesic properties have been known for many years, but up till the past decade, it has yet to find its place in analgesic regimens. There has been strong evidence suggesting the opioid-sparing properties of ketamine reduce the total consumption of opioids and their side effects, such as nausea, vomiting, and ileus [29, 30]. Ketamine acts as a non-competitive antagonist at NMDA receptors, producing its classical effects such as dissociation and hallucination. Still, the analgesic dose of 0.5 mg/kg rarely causes these. [31] Ketamine blocks signals from the ascending spinothalamic reticular pathways at the spinal level, reducing pain perception. Various other unknown mechanisms of action, such as magnesium channel blockade and phosphorylation of NMDA receptors, have been under research.

The parenteral route is the most widely used method of administration. Off-label uses such as infiltration, intranasal, nebulization, adjuvant to local anaesthetics in various regional procedures, and topical as a patch are not that popular. The ASA recommendations also suggest the usage of ketamine as part of a multimodal analgesia regimen in major thoracic and abdominal surgeries [15]. Wide dose ranges are quoted in the literature, starting from 0.5 mg/kg bolus and followed by an infusion of 10 μg/kg/min which can be titrated to the clinical effect. Notable adverse effects include an increase in blood pressure, arrhythmias, worsening of heart failure in patients with ischemic heart disease, increased skeletal muscle tone, and seizure-like activity, neurological symptoms such as hallucinations, anxiety, confusion, depression, respiratory symptoms including increased mucosal secretions, laryngospasm, etc. Ketamine is, as such, contraindicated in patients in whom an increase in blood pressure is detrimental, such as coronary artery disease, valvular heart defects, abdominal aortic aneurysm; also contraindicated in patients with increased intracranial pressure, severe hepatic, and renal dysfunction in whom there might be a delay in elimination of the drug [32].

5.3.2.4 α_2 Agonists

α_2 agonists such as dexmedetomidine and clonidine provide analgesia at peripheral, spinal, and supra-spinal levels based on the activation of postsynaptic α_2 receptors in the locus coeruleus of the brain stem and the spinal cord. [9] Both these drugs reduce the sympathetic tone causing bradycardia and hypotension and reduce opioid and anaesthetic requirements if used in the intraoperative period [33].Dexmedetomidine is relatively more selective at α_2 receptors with an α_2: α_1 activity of 1620:1 in comparison with clonidine with α_2: α_1 activity of 220:1, making it eight times more specific than clonidine. This is responsible for more effective sedation and analgesia produced by dexmedetomidine than clonidine [33]. Sedation with an easily arousable state upon stimulation, also called 'conscious sedation', is a characteristic feature of dexmedetomidine sedation, making it a highly recommended drug in any painful procedures which require sedation but not general anaesthesia.

Various routes of administration have been utilized in the literature, such as intranasal, parenteral, and perineural, in regional blocks as adjuvant and in neuraxial, both epidural and intrathecal. They are excellent adjuvants when used with local anaesthetics, causing significant prolongation in the nerve blockade in a dose-dependent manner without any significant adverse effects. ASA committee recommendations also strongly suggest the addition of clonidine or dexmedetomidine as an adjuvant to local anaesthetics to aid in prolongation of the effect if necessary [15]. A meta-analysis comparing fentanyl and dexmedetomidine as an adjuvant in spinal anaesthesia also proved that patients who received dexmedetomidine were pain-free for a longer duration with a similar amount of hypotension and bradycardia as that of fentanyl, without pruritus and vomiting [34].

Dexmedetomidine is administered as a standard bolus dose of 1 μg /kg over 10 min, followed by 0.3–0.7 μg/kg/h infusion for procedural sedation. A dose range of 0.5–1 mg/kg is used as an adjuvant in peripheral nerve blocks [35]. Most commonly encountered adverse effects include hypotension, bradycardia, and sometimes initial hypertension due to postsynaptic activation of receptors. There are, as such, no notable contraindications to dexmedetomidine, but it should be used cautiously in patients who might not tolerate such hemodynamic changes as in ischemic heart disease, heart failure, etc. [36]

5.3.2.5 Magnesium Sulphate

There has been a rapid increase in $MgSO_4$ usage in anaesthesia for the last decade. It has been classically used for a long time for the prevention of seizures in pre-eclampsia and as an anti-arrhythmic agent. It acts as a natural antagonist to Ca^{2+}, expressing the role of calcium channel blockers. It also acts as an antagonist at NMDA receptors, which prevent central sensitization in response to nociception and reduce hypersensitivity [37]. $MgSO_4$ had a big comeback into anaesthesia practice due to continuous recommendations of multimodal analgesia, guidelines with a bundle of recommendations such as Enhanced Recovery after Surgery (ERAS) and Procedure Specific Postoperative Pain Management (PROSPECT) guidelines.

The latest literature proves beyond doubt that $MgSO_4$ has antinociceptive effects, which can reduce perioperative opioid requirements even though there was wide variation in the dosage used [38]. A dose range of 30–50 mg/kg bolus followed by an infusion of 5–25 mg/kg/h was quoted in the literature. Other effects of $MgSO_4$ include improvement in microcirculation, prevention of vasospasm, maternal and fetal neuroprotection, potentiate nondepolarizing neuromuscular blocking agents, and bronchodilation.

Toxicity is rare but fatal unless diagnosed and promptly treated. Serum magnesium levels of 4–6 meq/L can cause nausea and lethargy, along with reduced deep tendon reflexes and hypotension.

At 6–10 meq/L, there can be bradycardia, absent deep tendon reflexes, prolonged PR interval, and increased QRS duration. At >10 meq/L, there can be coma, paralysis, respiratory failure, complete heart block, and cardiac arrest. Strict monitoring with discontinuation of the infusion and intravenous calcium is the treatment of choice.

5.3.2.6 Antiepileptic Drugs

Antiepileptic drugs such as gabapentin, pregabalin, clonazepam, carbamazepine, oxcarbazepine, topiramate, etc., are used widely in the treatment of neuropathic pain and chronic pain conditions such as fibromyalgia [39]. Gabapentin and pregabalin, called gabapentinoids, even though structurally similar to GABA, don't adhere to GABA receptors or don't have anything to do with them [40]. They have a high affinity for voltage-gated Ca^{2+} channels and prevent the release of excitatory mediators which increases the concentration of inhibitory mediators such as GABA [41]. Gabapentin is available in 100 mg, 300 mg, and 400 mg oral formulations and is prescribed in the dose range of 300 mg/day to 1200 mg/day. Pregabalin is started at 50 mg once at bedtime and can be increased up to 300 mg once daily. Common side effects include dizziness, sedation, ataxia, nausea, vomiting, diplopia, and life-threatening complications such as allergic reactions, angioedema, and with-drawl seizures can be seen rarely [40].

Oxcarbazepine and carbamazepine are the drugs of choice in the management of trigeminal neuralgia. These drugs block voltage-gated sodium channels, inhibiting action potential and stabilizing cell membranes in hyperexcitable neurons [41]. Carbamazepine is available in 100 mg, 200 mg, 300 mg, and 400 mg tablets. It is prescribed at 800–1200 mg/day up to a maximum of 1600 mg/day. Notable side effects include dizziness, ataxia, nausea, vomiting, hepatotoxicity, suicidal ideation, and hyponatremia. USFDA has issued a black box warning regarding agranulocytosis, a rare but severe side effect in these patients [42]. It is contraindicated in patients with bone marrow depression or documented hypersensitivity to other tricyclic antidepressants [42].

Topiramate is another antiepileptic drug with proven efficacy in the treatment of radicular pain and diabetic neuropathy [43]. It blocks AMPA (alpha-amino-3-hydroxy-5-methyl-4-isooxazole-propionic acid) gated sodium channels and also positively modulates GABA receptors, leading to antiepileptic activity, analgesia, as well as mood stabilization [44]. Common side effects, include CNS symptoms such as paraesthesia, tiredness, memory and concentration difficulties, endocrine and metabolic disturbances, suicidal ideation, ataxia, and worsening of glaucoma [44].

5.3.2.7 Antidepressants

Tricyclic antidepressants (TCA) such as amitriptyline and selective norepinephrine reuptake inhibitors such as duloxetine are being used in the management of neuropathic pain. They are also recommended prophylactically in patients with tension-type headaches and migraine [25]. Both these drugs cause inhibition in the reuptake of two primary neurotransmitters, serotonin and norepinephrine, resulting in the enhancement of descending inhibitory pathways in CNS related to pain. Also, TCA has anticholinergic, antihistaminic, and other effects, such as NMDA antagonism. Amitriptyline is available as 25 mg and 50 mg oral tablets (maximum daily dose 150 mg) and duloxetine as 60 mg and 120 mg tablets (maximum daily dose 120 mg). TCA can cause altered sensorium, arrhythmias, constipation, dry mouth, headache, reduced libido, orthostatic hypotension, and difficulty in urination [25]. Duloxetine causes nausea, vomiting, dizziness, hypertension, and suicidal ideation, for which regular monitoring is warranted [25].

5.3.2.8 Herbal Medication

Complementary and alternative medicine (CAM) strategies, including a wide range of therapies such as herbal medications such as ginger, turmeric, and capsaicin, were traditionally used for pain management after surgery in many countries. Many patients are under the assumption that these remedies are safe and natural methods to avoid the side effects of pharmacological agents. Still, most of them have active compounds that can produce a wide range of drug interactions [45]. The active components of ginger are called gingerols and traditionally have been used for the treatment of musculoskeletal pain, cold, motion sickness, swelling, arthritis, and nausea. It can produce side effects such as arrhythmias and sedation and increases bleeding time by preventing thromboxane synthesis [45].

Turmeric has an active compound called curcumin, which can regulate various cytokines such as IL-6, tumour necrosis factor - α (TNF - α), and interferons, leading to anti-inflammatory action [45]. Though it is being used widely for various autoimmune diseases such as rheumatoid arthritis, multiple sclerosis, and inflammatory bowel disease, it has been shown to increase bleeding time when used along with other antiplatelet medication [45]. Capsaicin is a chilly pepper extract with agonistic action at transient receptor potential cation channel type V 1 receptor (TRPV—1), leading to analgesic properties. The effect is particularly mentioned as 'defunctionalization' which is described as initial intense stinging, burning hyperalgesia followed by decreased sensitivity to noxious stimulation at 4–16 weeks after application [45]. Further research is required for validating these agents in perioperative practice for analgesia.

5.4 Conclusion

A wide variety of analgesic medications are available at the disposal of anaesthesiologists for the management of analgesia in the perioperative period. The choice of drug, dose, timing, and combination has to be selected based on the patient profile, surgery, type of pain, and the possible side effects. Multimodal analgesia has been a standard recommendation throughout the literature. It has proven to improve perioperative outcomes and reduce patient complications and hospital stays, aligning with the fast track and ERAS protocols. Judicious and evidence-based institutional pain management protocols must be established for each surgery to avoid complications.

Potential Conflicts of Interest None

References

1. Raja SN, Carr DB, Cohen M, Finnerup NB, Flor H, Gibson S, et al. The revised International Association for the Study of Pain definition of pain: concepts, challenges, and compromises. Pain [Internet]. 2020;161(9) Available from: https://www.ncbi.nlm.nih.gov/pmc/articles/PMC7680716/:1976.
2. Rachel H, Hendrix JM, Kramer J. Postoperative pain control. 2024 Jan 30. In: StatPearls [Internet]. Treasure Island: StatPearls Publishing; 2024. PMID: 31335018.
3. Gan TJ. Poorly controlled postoperative pain: prevalence, consequences, and prevention. J Pain Research [Internet]. 2017;10(1):2287–98. Available from: https://www.ncbi.nlm.nih.gov/pmc/articles/PMC5626380/
4. Vaurio LE, Sands LP, Wang Y, Mullen EA, Leung JM. Postoperative delirium: the importance of pain and pain management. Anesth Analg. 2006;102(4):1267–73.
5. Richebé P, Capdevila X, Rivat C. Persistent postsurgical pain pathophysiology and preventative pharmacologic considerations. Anesthesiology. 2018;129(3):590–607. Available from: https://anesthesiology.pubs.asahq.org/article.aspx?articleid=2681077
6. Lynch EP, Lazor MA, Gellis JE, Orav J, Goldman L, Marcantonio ER. The impact of postoperative pain on the development of postoperative delirium. Anesth Analg. 1998;86(4):781–5.
7. Robinson TN, Raeburn CD, Tran ZV, Angles EM, Brenner LA, Moss M. Postoperative delirium in the elderly: risk factors and outcomes. Ann Surg. 2009;249(1):173–8.
8. Blichfeldt-Eckhardt MR. From acute to chronic postsurgical pain: the significance of the acute pain response. Danish Med J [Internet]. 2018;65(3):B5326. Available from: https://pubmed.ncbi.nlm.nih.gov/29510808/
9. Pyati S, Gan TJ. Perioperative pain management. CNS Drugs. 2007;21(3):185–211.
10. Anekar AA, Cascella M, Hendrix JM. WHO analgesic ladder [Internet]. National Library of medicine. Treasure Island: StatPearls Publishing; 2023. Available from: https://www.ncbi.nlm.nih.gov/books/NBK554435/
11. Taylor A, McLeod G. Basic pharmacology of local anaesthetics. BJA Education [Internet]. 2020;20(2):34–41. Available from: https://www.bjaed.org/article/S2058-5349(19)30152-0/fulltext
12. Becker DE, Reed KL. Local anesthetics: review of pharmacological considerations. Anesthesia Progress [Internet]. 2012;59(2):90–102. Available from: https://www.ncbi.nlm.nih.gov/pmc/articles/PMC3403589/

13. Mahajan A, Derian A. Local anesthetic toxicity [Internet]. PubMed. Treasure Island: StatPearls Publishing; 2020. Available from: https://www.ncbi.nlm.nih.gov/books/NBK499964/
14. Neal JM, Neal EJ, Weinberg GL. American Society of Regional Anesthesia and Pain Medicine Local Anesthetic Systemic Toxicity checklist: 2020 version. Reg Anesth Pain Med. 2020. Nov 4;rapm-2020-101986;46:81.
15. Chou R, Gordon DB, de Leon-Casasola OA, Rosenberg JM, Bickler S, Brennan T, et al. Management of postoperative pain: a clinical practice guideline from the American Pain Society, the American Society of Regional Anesthesia and Pain Medicine, and the American Society of Anesthesiologists' Committee on Regional Anesthesia, Executive Committee, and Administrative Council. J Pain [Internet]. 2016;17(2):131–57. Available from: https://www.jpain.org/article/S1526-5900(15)00995-5/fulltext
16. Dhaliwal A, Gupta M. Physiology, Opioid receptor [Internet]. PubMed. Treasure Island: StatPearls Publishing; 2023. Available from: https://www.ncbi.nlm.nih.gov/books/NBK546642/
17. Lambert DG. Opioids and opioid receptors; understanding pharmacological mechanisms as a key to therapeutic advances and mitigation of the misuse crisis. BJA Open 2023;6:100141–1.
18. Algera MH, Kamp J, van der Schrier R, van Velzen M, Niesters M, Aarts L, et al. Opioid-induced respiratory depression in humans: a review of pharmacokinetic–pharmacodynamic modelling of reversal. Br J Anaesth [Internet]. 2019;122(6):e168–79. Available from: https://www.bjanaesthesia.org/article/S0007-0912(19)30008-X/fulltext
19. Schiller EY, Mechanic OJ. Opioid overdose [Internet]. National Library of Medicine. 2023; Available from: https://www.ncbi.nlm.nih.gov/books/NBK470415/
20. Miotto K, Cho AK, Khalil MA, Blanco K, Sasaki JD, Rawson R. Trends in tramadol: pharmacology, metabolism, and misuse. Anesth Analg [Internet]. 2017;124(1):44–51. Available from: https://www.ingentaconnect.com/content/wk/ane/2017/00000124/00000001/art00010
21. Lee SJ, Choi SJ, In CB, Sung TY. Effects of tramadol on emergence agitation after general anesthesia for nasal surgery. Medicine. 2019;98(10):e14763.
22. Wang X, Narayan SW, Penm J, Patanwala AE. Efficacy and safety of Tapentadol immediate release for acute pain. Clin J Pain. 2020;1:399.
23. Chen Q, Chen E, Qian X. A narrative review on perioperative pain management strategies in enhanced recovery pathways—the past, present and future. J Clin Med. 2021;10(12):2568.
24. Ghlichloo I, Gerriets V. Nonsteroidal anti-inflammatory drugs (NSAIDs) [Internet]. PubMed. Treasure Island: StatPearls Publishing; 2023. Available from: https://www.ncbi.nlm.nih.gov/books/NBK547742/

25. Queremel Milani DA, Davis DD. Pain management medications [Internet]. PubMed. Treasure Island: StatPearls Publishing; 2022. Available from: https://pubmed.ncbi.nlm.nih.gov/32809527/
26. Zarghi A, Arfaei S. Selective COX-2 inhibitors: a review of their structure-activity relationships. IJPR [Internet]. 2011;10(4):655–83. Available from: https://pubmed.ncbi.nlm.nih.gov/24250402/
27. Craig M, Jeavons R, Probert J, Benger J. Randomised comparison of intravenous paracetamol and intravenous morphine for acute traumatic limb pain in the emergency department. Emerg Med J [Internet]. 2011;29(1):37–9. Available from: https://emj.bmj.com/content/29/1/37
28. Agrawal S, Khazaeni B. Acetaminophen toxicity [Internet]. National Library of Medicine. StatPearls Publishing; 2023. Available from: https://www.ncbi.nlm.nih.gov/books/NBK441917/
29. Bell RF, Dahl JB, Moore RA, Kalso E. Peri-operative ketamine for acute post-operative pain: a quantitative and qualitative systematic review (Cochrane review). Acta Anaesthesiol Scand. 2005;49(10):1405–28.
30. Zhou L, Yang H, Hai Y, Cheng Y. Perioperative low-dose ketamine for postoperative pain management in spine surgery: a systematic review and meta-analysis of randomized controlled trials. Han F, editor. Pain Research and Management. 2022;2022:1–20.
31. Mion G, Villevieille T. Ketamine pharmacology: an update (pharmacodynamics and molecular aspects, recent findings). CNS Neurosci Therap [Internet]. 2013;19(6):370–80. Available from: http://www.thblack.com/links/RSD/CNSNeurosciTher2013_19_370_Pharmacology.pdf
32. Rosenbaum SB, Palacios JL. Ketamine [Internet]. Nih.gov. StatPearls Publishing; 2024. Available from: https://www.ncbi.nlm.nih.gov/books/NBK470357/
33. Gertler R, Brown HC, Mitchell DH, Silvius EN. Dexmedetomidine: a novel sedative-analgesic agent. Baylor Univ Med Cent Proc. 2001;14(1):13–21.
34. Sun S, Wang J, Bao N, Chen Y, Wang J. Comparison of dexmedetomidine and fentanyl as local anesthetic adjuvants in spinal anesthesia: a systematic review and meta-analysis of randomized controlled trials. Drug Des Devel Ther. 2017;11:3413–24.
35. Koyyalamudi V, Sen S, Patil S, Creel JB, Cornett EM, Fox CJ, et al. Adjuvant agents in regional anesthesia in the ambulatory setting. Curr Pain Headache Rep. 2017;21(1):6.
36. Reel B, Maani CV. Dexmedetomidine [Internet]. PubMed. Treasure Island: StatPearls Publishing; 2023. Available from: https://www.ncbi.nlm.nih.gov/books/NBK513303/
37. Tramer MR, Schneider J, Marti RA, Rifat K. Role of magnesium sulfate in postoperative analgesia. Anesthesiology. 1996;84(2):340–7.
38. Albrecht E, Kirkham KR, Liu SS, Brull R. Peri-operative intravenous administration of magnesium sulphate and postoperative pain: a meta-analysis. Anaesthesia. 2012;68(1):79–90.

39. Wiffen PJ, Derry S, Moore RA, Aldington D, Cole P, Rice ASC, et al. Antiepileptic drugs for neuropathic pain and fibromyalgia—an overview of Cochrane reviews. The Cochrane database of systematic reviews [Internet]. 2013;2013(11):CD010567. Available from: https://www.ncbi.nlm.nih.gov/pubmed/24217986
40. Yasaei R, Katta S, Saadabadi A. Gabapentin [Internet]. PubMed. Treasure Island: StatPearls Publishing; 2024. Available from: https://www.ncbi.nlm.nih.gov/books/NBK493228/
41. Gambeta E, Chichorro JG, Zamponi GW. Trigeminal neuralgia: an overview from pathophysiology to pharmacological treatments. Mol Pain. 2020;16:174480692090189.
42. Maan JS, Saadabadi A. Carbamazepine [Internet]. Nih.gov: StatPearls Publishing; 2023. Available from: https://www.ncbi.nlm.nih.gov/books/NBK482455/
43. Muehlbacher M, Nickel MK, Kettler C, Tritt K, Lahmann C, Leiberich PK, et al. Topiramate in treatment of patients with chronic low Back pain. Clin J Pain. 2006;22(6):526–31.
44. Fariba K, Saadabadi A. Topiramate [Internet]. PubMed. Treasure Island: StatPearls Publishing; 2020. Available from: https://www.ncbi.nlm.nih.gov/books/NBK554530/
45. Jahromi B, Pirvulescu I, Candido KD, Knezevic NN. Herbal medicine for pain management: efficacy and drug interactions. Pharmaceutics [Internet]. 2021;13(2):251. Available from: https://www.ncbi.nlm.nih.gov/pmc/articles/PMC7918078/

Methods of Analgesia

6

Sadik Mohammed and Anita Chouhan

Abstract

Pain is the most common reason for a patient to seek medical advice. The management of acute pain is crucial as inadequate/inappropriate management has been found to be associated with increased morbidity. Opioids have been the mainstay of analgesic regime for management of acute pain. They can be administered via various routes including intravenous, epidural, intrathecal, nerve block, etc. This chapter provides an overview of patient-controlled analgesia, neuraxial block, and peripheral nerve block techniques used for managing acute pain.

Keywords

Acute pain · Neuraxial analgesia · Patient-controlled analgesia · Pain management · Peripheral nerve blocks

S. Mohammed (✉) · A. Chouhan
Department of Anesthesiology and Critical Care, All India Institute of Medical Sciences (AIIMS) Jodhpur, Jodhpur, India
e-mail: mohammeds@aiimsjodhpur.edu.in; chouhana@aiimsjodhpur.edu.in

P. Ahluwalia (ed.), *Handbook of Perioperative Analgesia*,
https://doi.org/10.1007/978-981-96-7822-8_6

Key Points

- PCA allows patients to self-administer a predetermined dose of analgesic, typically via an IV pump. It is programmed with a lockout interval to prevent overdose. It improves patient autonomy and satisfaction and provides pain relief tailored to immediate needs.
- Neuraxial blocks consist of an injection of analgesics near the spinal cord within the epidural or subarachnoid space. It provides superior pain control, reduced opioid consumption, and early ambulation.
- Peripheral nerve block provides targeted analgesia by injecting local anesthetics near a specific nerve or group of nerves. It has been an effective method for site-specific pain relief with reduced need for systemic opioids and improved recovery.

"I put it to you that the relief of severe, unrelenting pain would come at the top of a list of basic human rights." M. J. Cousins

6.1 Introduction

Pain is defined as "an unpleasant sensory and emotional experience associated with, or resembling that associated with actual or potential tissue damage." [1] The World Health Organization (WHO) and the International Association for the Study of Pain (IASP) acknowledge that alleviating pain is a basic human right [2]. Pain is typically categorized into three types: "acute pain" (associated with trauma, labor, and both surgical and post-surgical pain), cancer pain, and chronic non-cancer pain.

The management of acute pain is crucial as inadequate/inappropriate management has been found to be associated with increased morbidity. It negatively affects quality of life and functional recovery and is an independent risk factor for persistent pain and long-term opioid use [3]. Opioids have been the mainstay of analgesic regime for management of acute pain. However, opioid related side effects and risk of opioid dependence emphasizes the need for alternative, analgesic techniques which includes neuraxial (epidural/intrathecal) techniques, peripheral nerve blocks, use of non-opioid medications, etc. This chapter will explore these analgesic methods, examining their mechanisms, applications, benefits, and potential risks, with the aim of providing a comprehensive understanding of how these techniques contribute to effective pain management strategies. Non-opioid adjuvants are discussed in chapter on "Drugs for acute pain management."

6.2 Patient-Controlled Analgesia

Since 1971, patient-controlled analgesia (PCA) has been used to enhance pain management, with the first commercially available PCA pump introduced in 1976. The purpose of PCA is to provide effective pain relief by allowing patients to self-administer a preset dose of medication on-demand with the push of a button, according to their preferred dosage and timing, thereby enhancing the patient autonomy and comfort. Each dose can be given alone or combined with a continuous background infusion of medication. PCA is used to manage acute, chronic, postoperative, and labor-related pain [4]. Medications can be delivered intravenously (IV), epidurally, via a peripheral nerve catheter, or trans dermally [5, 6].

PCA has been shown to be more effective for pain control compared to non-patient-administered or intermittent analgesic injections, leading to greater patient satisfaction, increased perception of situational control, lower anxiety and depressive symptoms, and increased control over pain relief [7, 8]. Additional benefits include avoiding the need for injections, experiencing immediate pain relief and lesser dependency on nursing staff thereby enhancing overall satisfaction with pain management [9]. Despite these advantages, PCA has been linked to negative experiences such as distrust of the PCA pump, concerns about overdose or addiction, and potential adverse effects like oversedation and respiratory depression [10]. Adherence to stringent clinical guidelines is crucial to mitigate these adverse outcomes [11].

6.2.1 Equipment and Operation

The administration of PCA involves choosing the appropriate route, medication, and pump type.

Routes: PCA can be administered via an intravenous (IV) catheter, epidural catheter, indwelling nerve catheter, or iontophoretic transdermal system.

Pumps: A range of PCA pumps are available, but all share key features such as a locking device, medication chamber, programming screen, and patient button (Fig. 6.1). The physician manages the infusion rate, bolus volume, maximum allowable hourly dose, and lockout interval. The patient, however, controls the button that delivers a bolus dose of drug. The lockout time is a crucial safety feature of PCA that prevents unintentional overdose, ensuring patient safety. Furthermore, if a patient receives excessive drug known to cause sedation, the resulting sedation will naturally limit further self-administration [12]. For IV PCA, the medication line is connected to a fluid infusion line.

Medications: Commonly used medications include opioids and local anesthetics. Opioids are typically used alone for IV PCA (Table 6.1) or combined with local anesthetics for epidural catheter or peripheral nerve catheter PCA (Table 6.2). Opioids include pure Mu opioid receptor agonists (morphine, fentanyl, hydromorphone, sufentanil, alfentanil, and remifentanil), Mu opioid receptor agonist-antagonists (butorphanol, nalbuphine, pentazocine), and partial Mu opioid receptor agonists (buprenorphine, dezocine). Among these, morphine remains the gold standard for IV PCA [13]. Other medications like ketamine, naloxone, clonidine, magnesium, and ketorolac may be added to IV PCA to improve pain control and reduce side effects. However, opioids and local anesthetics remain the core of PCA therapy [13]. Local anesthetics, such as bupivacaine, levobupivacaine, and ropivacaine, with or without adjuvants, are primarily used for epidural catheters and indwelling nerve catheters PCA.

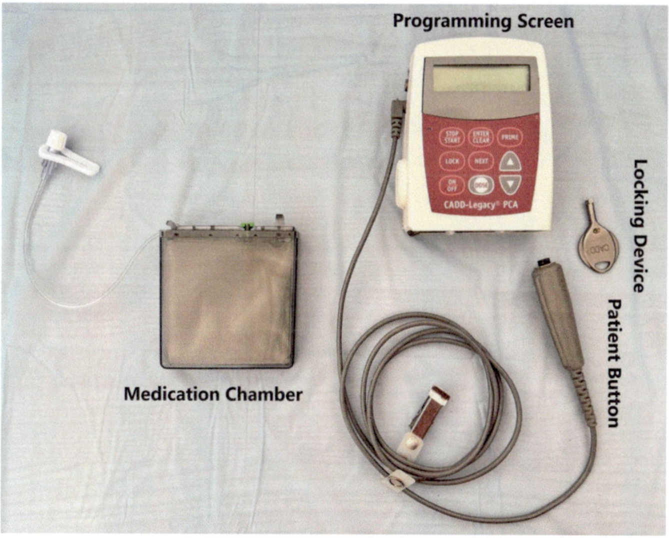

Fig. 6.1 PCA pump showing different parts (programing screen, medication chamber, patient button). (CADD-Legacy® PCA, Model 6300, Smith Medical ASD, Inc., St. Paul, MN 55112, USA)

Table 6.1 Setting of intravenous patient-controlled analgesia (PCA)

Analgesic	Bolus dose	Lockout period (minutes)	Basal infusion rate
Morphine	1–2 mg	5–10	≤0.5 mg/h
Fentanyl	10–50 μg	5–10	≤50 μg/h
Sufentanil	4–6 μg	5–10	≤5 μg/h
Remifentanil	0.5 μg/kg	2	NA
Piritramide	0.75–1.5 mg	5–10	≤0.5 mg/h
Hydromorphone	0.25–0.5 mg	5–10	≤0.4 mg/h
Tramadol	10–20 mg	5–10	≤10 mg/h

Table 6.2 Setting of patient-controlled epidural analgesia (PCEA) and peripheral nerve catheter PCA

Purpose	Drug and concentration	Basal infusion rate (mL)	Demand dose (mL)	Lockout period (minutes)
Labor Epidural Analgesia	Bupivacaine 0.0625% to 0.125% + Fentanyl 1-2 μg/mL	5–10	3–5	10–15
	Ropivacaine 0.08% to 0.1% + Fentanyl 1-2 μg/mL	5–10	3–5	10–15
Lumber Epidural for Infra-umbilical Surgeries	Bupivacaine 0.0625% + Fentanyl 5 μg/mL	4	4	10
	Bupivacaine 0.125% + Fentanyl 5 μg/mL ± Clonidine 0.75 μg/mL	4	3	10
	Bupivacaine 0.0625% + Hydromorphone 10 μg/mL	4	4	10
	Bupivacaine 0.0625% + Clonidine 1 μg/mL	4	4	10
Interscalene or infraclavicular brachial plexus	Ropivacaine 0.2%	6–8	2–4	20
Sub-gluteal or Popliteal Sciatic	Ropivacaine 0.2%	5–8	3–5	20–60

6.3 Neuraxial Analgesia

Neuraxial analgesia involves administering local anesthetics and/or opioids in subanesthetic doses to the neuraxis for effective, long-lasting pain relief. It can be administered through a single injection into the epidural or subarachnoid space, via intermittent injections or continuous infusion through an epidural catheter, or by patient-controlled epidural analgesia (PCEA) using a catheter. The use of subarachnoid catheters for acute pain is uncommon. It is commonly used for intraoperative analgesia, postoperative pain, and chronic cancer pain. This technique has been shown to offer highly effective pain relief [14]. Additionally, it may provide benefits beyond pain relief. Neuraxial opioids are commonly used during labor and delivery, but they are also applied in procedures such as laparotomies, thoracotomies, cardiac surgery, and lower limb arthroplasty [15–19]. One of the key advantages of epidural analgesia is seen in patients with preexisting respiratory conditions undergoing abdominal surgery [20].

A key factor in choosing patients for neuraxial analgesia is their coagulation status, especially if they are taking antiplatelet or anticoagulant medications. Understanding coagulation issues is crucial to reducing the risk of intraspinal bleeding and spinal hematomas, which can cause serious neurological damage [21].

6.3.1 Anatomy

The spinal cord extends from the brainstem and terminates at the conus medullaris, with the filum terminale and cauda equina extending further. In adults, the spinal cord ends at L1-L2; in infants, it can end at L3 due to differential growth rates. Three meninges surround the spinal cord: the pia mater (innermost), arachnoid mater, and dura mater (outermost). Cerebrospinal fluid (CSF) resides in the subarachnoid space between the pia and arachnoid mater. The arachnoid mater serves as a major barrier to drug passage into and out of the CSF [22].

The epidural space, external to the dura mater, is bounded by the posterior longitudinal ligament, pedicles, and ligamentum flavum, and contains nerve roots, fat, areolar tissue, lymphatics, and Batson's venous plexus. The ligamentum flavum varies in thickness and proximity to the dura across vertebral levels [22].

6.3.2 Mechanism of Action

Neuraxial analgesia works by blocking sensory, motor, and sympathetic nerve fibers through the administration of local anesthetics and/or opioids.

The pharmacologic properties of various opioids determine their speed of onset, duration of action, and side effect profile (Table 6.3). The lipid solubility of a drug is a key factor in its effectiveness when administered via the neuraxial route. Morphine, being hydrophilic, has a slower onset of analgesia, a longer duration of action, the ability to provide pain relief across a broader dermatomal range, and carries a risk of delayed respiratory depression. In contrast, fentanyl is lipophilic, resulting in a rapid onset, a shorter duration of action, more localized pain relief, and a reduced risk of delayed respiratory depression. Hydrophilic opioids like morphine, when introduced into the epidural or subarachnoid space, tend to remain in the cerebrospinal fluid (CSF) longer than lipophilic ones, allowing them to travel to the brain and affect respiratory centers hours after administration [23]. Opioids administered into the epidural space diffuse into surrounding tissues, including epidural fat and veins, reducing their availability to bind to opioid receptors and provide analgesia. Epidural opioids primarily exert their analgesic effects through two mechanisms: spinal and supraspinal or systemic pathways. Some opioids enter the

Table 6.3 Pharmacological characteristics of commonly used neuraxial opioids

Drug	Oil-water partition coefficient (lipophilicity)	Dose (μg)	Onset (min)	Duration (h)
Morphine	1.4	50–500	30–60	10–24
Fentanyl	816	10–50	5–10	0.5–2
Sufentanil	1727	2.5–12.5	3–6	1–3

cerebrospinal fluid (CSF) by diffusing through the spinal meninges, resulting in spinally mediated analgesia. Others are absorbed into the bloodstream and transported to the brainstem, where they contribute to supraspinal analgesia [24].

Local anesthetics used for neuraxial analgesia work by blocking nerve conduction. To achieve this form of analgesia, smaller doses and lower concentrations of local anesthetics are administered compared to those required for surgical anesthesia. This sensory blockade provides sufficient pain relief without significantly affecting motor function, allowing for the detection of complications. Additionally, analgesic doses of local anesthetics result in less disruption of sympathetic tone. Bupivacaine and ropivacaine are the most commonly used local anesthetics for epidural analgesia due to their preferential effect on sensory fibers over motor fibers (differential blockade) and their lower likelihood of causing tachyphylaxis (tolerance to local anesthetic effects).

For acute pain, neuraxial analgesia often combines opioids with local anesthetics, as their differing mechanisms of action work synergistically to provide enhanced pain relief with reduced doses and fewer side effects. Intrathecal (IT) meperidine is notable as it has both local anesthetic effects and opioid receptor-binding properties, making it suitable as a standalone agent for surgery. It induces spinal anesthesia similar in quality to that provided by conventional local anesthetics. Despite being less lipid-soluble than fentanyl, meperidine has a similar onset of action but a longer duration [25].

6.3.3 Benefits and Limitations

Subarachnoid or Intrathecal (Spinal): This technique involves the direct administration of opioids into the cerebrospinal fluid (CSF) for analgesia. Intrathecal (IT) opioids offer several advantages, including prolonged duration of action, the need for smaller doses to achieve equivalent analgesic effects, minimal vascular absorption, ease of intrathecal space access, minimal hemodynamic alterations, and the absence of motor blockade or sensory loss. However, potential side effects include mild respiratory depression, respiratory arrest, pruritus, generalized muscle rigidity, sedation, nystagmus, nausea and vomiting, epileptic seizures, myoclonus, urinary retention, hyperalgesia, neurotoxicity, and water retention [23].

Epidural: It involves administration of analgesics via an indwelling catheter placed in the epidural space. Although opioids may be used alone for providing effective postoperative analgesia, multiple studies have shown that analgesia is more effective when they are combined with lower concentration of local anesthetics. It has been considered to be the gold standard for providing labor analgesia and postoperative analgesia following various surgeries. The advantages and side effects are similar to intrathecal opioids.

6.3.4 Advancements in Neuraxial Analgesia

Recent advancements in neuraxial analgesia include:

Low-concentration anesthetic-opioid solutions: To reduce side effects while maintaining efficacy.

Patient-Controlled Epidural Analgesia (PCEA): Allows patients to self-administer predetermined doses of analgesics, improving pain management and patient satisfaction.

Automated boluses: Such as programmed intermittent or automated mandatory boluses, to maintain effective analgesia and reduce the need for manual adjustments.

6.3.5 Neuraxial Analgesia for Cancer Pain

Neuraxial analgesia is a valuable option for treating refractory cancer pain [26]. The most common approach involves the insertion of an intrathecal catheter for continuous opioid administration, often combined with local anesthetics and adjuvants such as clonidine. Percutaneous catheters, particularly when tunneled, can be maintained for extended periods with proper aseptic techniques and care. These catheters can also be used in home settings, provided adequate home care infrastructure is available [27].

6.3.6 Neuraxial Analgesia in Labor

Neuraxial analgesia, including epidural, spinal, and combined spinal-epidural (CSE) techniques, is widely utilized for labor analgesia [28]. This method involves the administration of local anesthetics and opioids into the epidural or subarachnoid space. Neuraxial techniques are favored for their effectiveness in relieving labor pain, improving maternal comfort, and reducing pain-induced complications such as hypertension and tachycardia. Although other adjuvants like epinephrine and clonidine are used to reduce the local anesthetic dose, opioids remain the primary agents due to their proven efficacy. Clonidine's use is limited by potential side effects, including hypotension.

6.4 Peripheral Nerve Blocks

Peripheral nerve blocks (PNBs) are effective means of providing surgical anesthesia and postoperative analgesia for many surgical procedures involving the upper and lower extremities as well as nonsurgical analgesia. In certain situations, PNBs offer distinct benefits over general or neuraxial anesthesia [29].

Advancements in nerve block equipment and techniques, along with the availability of various local anesthetics, have significantly enhanced the safety and effectiveness of PNBs. Beyond their role in providing anesthesia for surgeries and the use of indwelling catheters for extended nerve blocks, PNBs offer excellent pain relief for many upper extremity surgeries and traumas. Additionally, indwelling catheters are useful in promoting blood flow following limb reattachment surgeries or in patients with peripheral vascular disease.

Vasoconstrictors, typically epinephrine, can be added to local anesthetics to reduce drug absorption and extend the duration of action. A concentration between 1:200,000 and 1:400,000 is generally recommended. Ideally, epinephrine should be mixed with the anesthetic just before the block is administered. Commercial solutions containing epinephrine tend to have a lower pH, leading to a higher proportion of ionized drug molecules, which slows their ability to penetrate neural membranes and delays the onset of action. Other additives, such as steroids, clonidine, dexmedetomidine, opioids, and ketamine, have also been noted to enhance or extend the effects of local anesthetic. Liposomal bupivacaine, which provides a slow release of the anesthetic, is FDA-approved for facial plane and interscalene nerve blocks. However, its advantage over single-dose long-acting anesthetics or continuous catheters for providing prolonged blocks has not been consistently proven [30].

While each type of block comes with its own specific risks and benefits, common complications associated with PNBs include local anesthetic toxicity, nerve injury, accidental neuraxial block, and unintentional injection of local anesthetics into blood vessels resulting in systemic toxicity.

6.4.1 Type of Nerve Block

Single Injections—A single-injection nerve block, commonly referred to as a "single-shot" block, involves delivering a one-time dose of local anesthetic near a specific nerve or plexus to induce anesthesia or pain relief. The duration and intensity of the block are influenced by factors such as the dose, concentration, and pharmacological properties of the chosen anesthetic, with effects ranging from less than an hour to over 24 h.

Continuous nerve block—A continuous nerve block involves the ongoing infusion of local anesthetic through a catheter positioned near a peripheral nerve or plexus, providing prolonged anesthesia or pain relief. This technique is effective for both inpatient and outpatient settings, particularly for patients needing extended pain management. By minimizing pain, opioid consumption, and related side effects, continuous nerve blocks enhance patient comfort and improve overall satisfaction, including better sleep quality.

6.4.2 Techniques for Localizing Nerves

Paresthesia Techniques—Paresthesia-seeking involves eliciting a tingling sensation by contacting a nerve with the needle. Though historically common, it can cause discomfort and potential nerve damage. Blunt beveled needles may push nerves aside with less risk of penetration, while sharp needles can cause more severe injuries if they penetrate. This technique has been largely replaced by more advanced methods but remains relevant in certain contexts.

Peripheral Nerve Stimulation—Peripheral nerve stimulator uses electrical currents to induce muscle contractions, aiding in nerve localization without patient feedback. A higher current initially helps identify the nerve, which is then confirmed with a lower current. This technique allows for better sedation and reduces reliance on patient responses.

Ultrasound Guidance—Ultrasound provides real-time imaging of nerves, the needle tip, and local anesthetic distribution, offering significant advantages over other methods. There are various techniques for performing regional blocks using ultrasound. Peripheral nerves are typically visualized in a short-axis view rather than a long-axis view. The needle can either be inserted within the plane of the ultrasound image (in-plane technique) or cross the plane of the image, appearing as an echogenic dot (out-of-plane technique). Research suggests that the key to successful outcomes in regional blocks lies in properly visualizing and identifying relevant structures—such as the peripheral nerve, needle tip, local anesthetic, and nearby anatomy—rather than the specific technique used.

6.4.3 Brachial Plexus Block

6.4.3.1 Anatomy

The brachial plexus arises from the anterior primary rami of the fifth to eighth cervical nerves (C5-C8) and the first thoracic nerve (T1), with occasional contributions from C4 and T2. After exiting

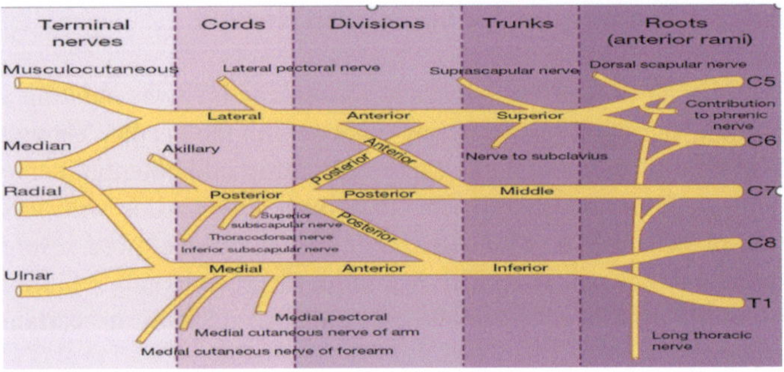

Fig. 6.2 Schematic diagram showing formation of Brachial plexus and its branches. (Adapted from www.google.com)

the intervertebral foramina, these nerves pass between the anterior and middle scalene muscles. The plexus is encased within a fascial sheath derived from the prevertebral fascia.

Within the interscalene space, the nerve roots combine to form three trunks: the superior (C5-C6), middle (C7), and inferior (C8-T1). As they reach the lateral edge of the first rib, each trunk divides into anterior and posterior divisions before continuing into the infraclavicular region. In this area, these divisions reorganize into three cords—lateral, posterior, and medial—named based on their position relative to the second part of the axillary artery. At the lateral border of the pectoralis minor muscle, the cords further branch into the peripheral nerves supplying the upper extremity (Fig. 6.2) [31].

6.4.4 Approaches for Brachial Plexus Block

6.4.4.1 Interscalene Block

Interscalene block targets the roots/trunks of the brachial plexus. The superior and middle trunks are blocked consistently; however, the inferior trunk (C8-T1) often spared, as it emerges much lower in the neck. Therefore, it can be used for surgeries that involve the distal clavicle, shoulder, and upper arm [32]. For the block, the patient is positioned supine with head turned away

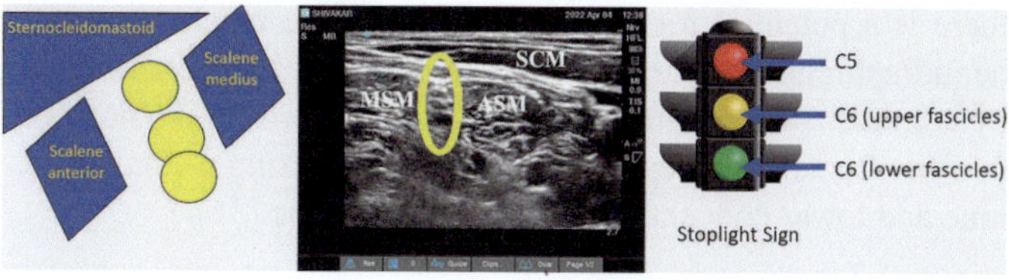

Fig. 6.3 Schematic diagram (left) and Sono anatomy (right) of brachial plexus at interscalene level showing typical "traffic light sign." (ASM Anterior Scalene Muscle; MSM Middle Scalene Muscle; SCM Sternocleidomastoid Muscle; C5 5th Cervical Root; C6 6th Cervical Root)

from the blocked side, and arm by the side of the body in a comfortable position.

A continuous interscalene brachial plexus block offers a superior option compared to a single-shot block, as it ensures prolonged pain relief, decreases overall postoperative morphine use, and lowers both dynamic and resting pain scores for up to 48 h, without raising the risk of complications [33].

6.4.4.2 Sono Anatomy

A high frequency linear ultrasound transducer placed in a transverse plane at the C6 vertebral level provides a short-axis view of the brachial plexus. The middle scalene muscle, anterior scalene muscle, sternocleidomastoid muscle, and brachial plexus are identified. The sono-anatomy has a "stoplight" appearance of the brachial plexus that refers typically to a monofascicular C5 and bifascicular C6 ventral rami aligned in a parallel fashion from superficial to deep (Fig. 6.3) [34]. An in-plane or out-of-plane approach can be used to advance the needle. Injection of a small volume of normal saline or local anesthetic confirms needle placement in the interscalene groove. A volume of 5–10 mL with an observation of spread of the local anesthetic along the roots ensure successful block, with minimal or no diaphragmatic paresis.

6.4.4.3 Side Effects and Complications

The interscalene block carries risks such as Horner syndrome, recurrent laryngeal nerve block, epidural or subarachnoid injection, vertebral artery injection, and pneumothorax. Additionally, there is a potential for transient phrenic nerve block, leading to hemidiaphragmatic paresis. However, this risk can be minimized by administering the interscalene injection lower in the neck (by performing selective upper trunk block) and using a smaller volume and lower concentration of local anesthetic [35].

6.4.4.4 Supraclavicular Block

The supraclavicular block is an effective technique for providing anesthesia and analgesia for the upper limb, making it suitable for surgical procedures, trauma management, chronic upper extremity pain, and vascular insufficiency. The brachial plexus at this level is compact, allowing for a rapid and reliable onset of anesthesia with a relatively small volume of local anesthetic. Traditionally, the block has not been considered to be an optimal choice for placement of catheters as mobility of the neck at this location carries a risk for catheter dislodgement.

6.4.4.5 Sono Anatomy

For this block, the patient is positioned supine with head turned away from the blocked side, and arm adducted against the body. A high-frequency (15–6 MHz) linear transducer placed just proximal to the supraclavicular fossa to obtain a supraclavicular view. The brachial plexus trunks and divisions are visualized clustered over the first rib, postero-lateral to the subclavian artery. The sono-anatomical appearance is often described as resembling a cluster or bunch of grapes (Fig. 6.4). Ultrasound guidance aids in identifying key structures, avoiding blood vessels, ensuring the proper distribution of local anesthetic, and recognizing as well as avoiding the pleura. The needle is advanced using an in-plane approach from lateral to medial direction. The first rib acts as a barrier to prevent the needle from reaching the pleural dome. After negative aspiration, a small test dose of local anesthetic is administered and the spread of the anesthetic around the brachial plexus is observed for correct placement of needle.

To accelerate the onset, the two-injection technique is employed, involving the administration of 10–15 mL of local

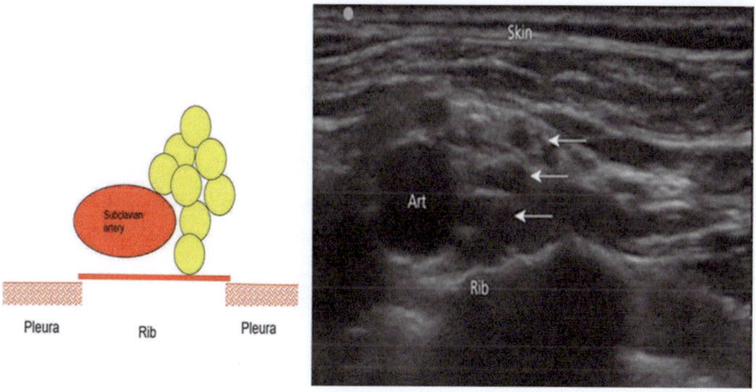

Fig. 6.4 Schematic diagram (left) and Sono anatomy (right) of brachial plexus at supraclavicular level showing typical "bunch of grapes appearance"

anesthetic at the "corner pocket" (formed by the subclavian artery, first rib, and brachial plexus) and an additional 10 mL at a more superficial site near the brachial plexus or, less frequently, among the nerves. This targeted approach offers the benefits of a faster onset and an extended duration of action. Alternatively, a single injection of 20–30 mL of local anesthetic at the "corner pocket" is a practical option, especially when the block is primarily intended for postoperative pain relief. This single-injection method is more time-efficient and minimizes needle manipulation.

6.4.4.6 Side Effects and Complications

Pneumothorax, manifested as cough, dyspnea, or pleuritic chest pain, has been the most common serious complication of a supraclavicular block (about a 1% incidence). Although ultrasound guidance helps reduce this risk, it does not eliminate it. Phrenic nerve blockade is a common occurrence, affecting approximately 50% of procedures, though it typically does not result in clinically significant symptoms. However, bilateral supraclavicular blocks are not advised due to the risk of bilateral pneumothorax or phrenic nerve paralysis. Similarly, patients with chronic obstructive pulmonary disease (COPD) may not be ideal candidates for this block [31].

6.4.4.7 Infraclavicular Block

The infraclavicular approach targets the brachial plexus at the level of the cords providing comprehensive anesthesia/analgesia covering the entire forearm and hand. It is advantageous for its stable catheter placement and minimal need for arm manipulation [36]. However, it requires deeper needle placement and careful technique due to the challenging visualization of the needle tip and neurovascular structures.

6.4.4.8 Sono Anatomy

The patient can be placed in either a supine or semi-recumbent position. Abducting the arm helps in aligning the neurovascular bundle for easier access. A high-frequency linear probe (5–15 MHz) is placed medial to the coracoid process and caudal to the clavicle in a transverse (short-axis) view. The axillary artery and vein can be visualized below the overlying pectoralis major and minor muscles. The lateral, medial, and posterior cords appear as hyperechoic structures with hypoechoic nerve fascicles on ultrasound (Fig. 6.5). Typically, the cords are positioned around

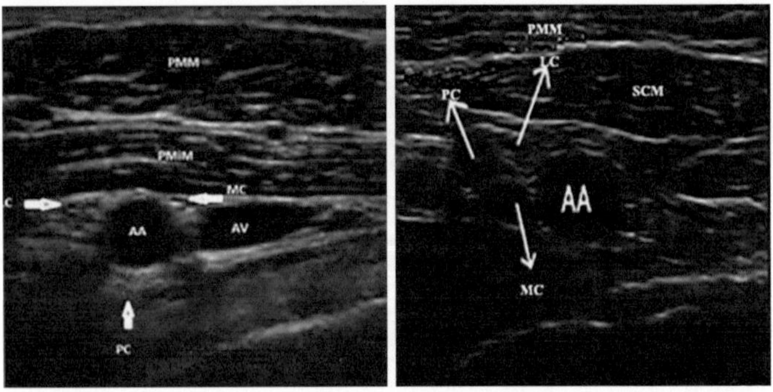

Fig. 6.5 Sono anatomy of brachial plexus at infraclavicular level showing arrangement of the cord in relation to the axillary artery in the lateral infraclavicular area (left) and medial (costoclavicular space) infraclavicular area (right). (PMM Pectoralis Major Muscle; PMiM Pectoralis Minor Muscle; SCM Subclavius Muscle; MC Medial Cord; LC Lateral Cord; PC Posterior Cord; AV Axillary Vein; AA Axillary Artery)

the axillary artery, with the posterior cord located at the 6 o'clock position, while the lateral and medial cords are variably situated near the 3 and 9 o'clock positions, respectively [36]. An in-plane approach typically from the lateral side of the probe is used with a 22-gauge, 5-cm needle. The needle is inserted at a steep angle and advanced until the tip is positioned posterior to the axillary artery. Injection of 20–30 mL of local anesthetic would achieve a complete block. The two most well documented injection techniques are the posterior cord injection and a triple-injection technique (LA is administered around each cord of the plexus). While the triple-injection method has a high success rate, it does not offer a significant advantage over the single posterior injection approach [37].

The costoclavicular approach to the infraclavicular brachial plexus block has recently been introduced as a medial (proximal) technique for accessing the cords [38]. In this approach, the brachial plexus lies more superficially compared to the traditional distal infraclavicular method. At this level, the cords are positioned closely together and distinct from the axillary artery, unlike the standard infraclavicular block, where the cords are more variably distributed around the artery and spaced farther apart (Fig. 6.5).

6.4.4.9 Side Effects and Complications

Although pneumothorax is a potential risk with the infraclavicular block, it remains low when proper technique, needle orientation, and guidance are used. Self-limiting side effects commonly associated with the supraclavicular block, such as hoarseness, Horner syndrome, and phrenic nerve paresis, may also occur with the infraclavicular block but are less frequent [39]. There is an increased risk of hematoma with conventional approach due to it being deep blocks in non-compressible locations.

6.4.4.10 Axillary Block

The axillary block is a widely used technique for providing anesthesia to the upper extremity and is particularly effective for surgeries involving the elbow and distal arm. It has traditionally faced challenges, particularly with the inconsistent blockade of the musculocutaneous nerve. However, the advent of ultrasound imaging has significantly improved the efficacy and precision of this block, allowing for better visualization and targeting of the musculocutaneous nerve.

The continuous axillary brachial plexus block has been successfully utilized, though it is not widely practiced. The use of axillary block catheters carries a relatively high risk of local inflammation and bacterial colonization [40].

6.4.5 Lumbosacral Plexus Block

6.4.5.1 Anatomy

The lumbosacral plexus (Fig. 6.6) is a network of nerves formed by the branches of spinal nerves from L1 to S4, providing motor and sensory functions to the lower limbs and pelvis. It is divided into two main parts: the lumbar plexus (L1-L4) and the sacral plexus (L4-S4). The lumbar plexus is located within the psoas major muscle and includes important nerves like the femoral nerve (L2-L4), which controls the anterior thigh muscles, and the obturator nerve (L2-L4), which controls the medial thigh. The lateral femoral cutaneous nerve (L2-L3) supplies sensation to the outer thigh, while smaller nerves like the iliohypogastric and ilioinguinal nerves (L1) provide sensation to the groin and lower abdomen.

The sacral plexus, situated on the front of the piriformis muscle, gives rise to the sciatic nerve (L4-S3), the largest nerve in the body, which supplies the posterior thigh and lower leg. Other branches include the superior and inferior gluteal nerves (L4-S2), which innervate the gluteal muscles, and the pudendal nerve (S2-S4), which controls the muscles of the pelvic floor [41].

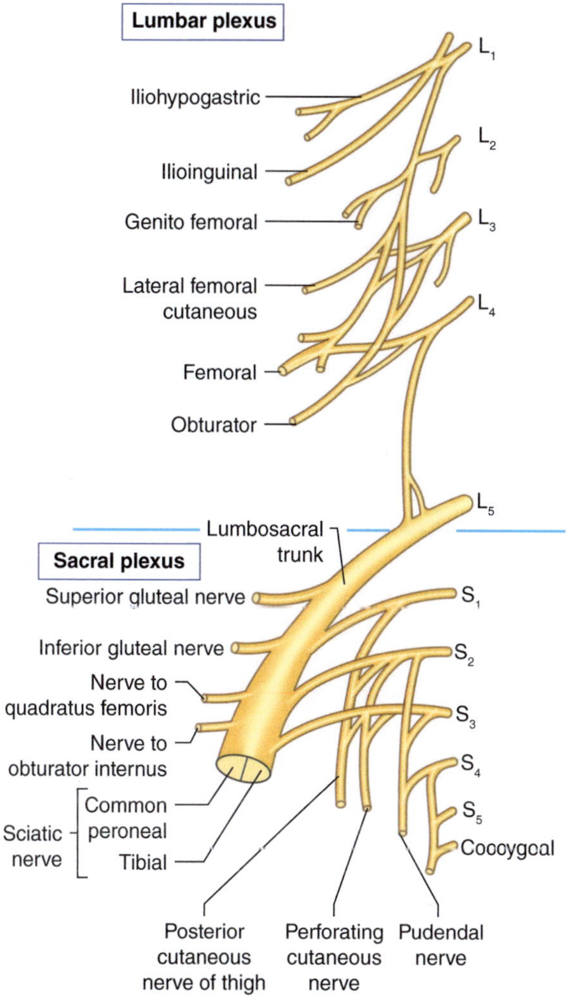

Fig. 6.6 Schematic diagram showing formation of Lumbosacral plexus and its branches. (Adapted from www.google.com)

6.4.6 Approaches to Lumbosacral Plexus Block

6.4.6.1 Lumbar Plexus Block

The lumbar plexus block, despite its effectiveness for hip and knee surgeries, has seen reduced adoption due to its complexity and potential complications arising from the deep location near critical structures like the epidural space and lumbar arteries. The lumbar plexus block is primarily used in surgeries involving the hip, femur, and knee. It provides effective analgesia by blocking the nerves supplying the anterior and medial portions of the thigh, as well as the knee joint. Continuous catheter can be placed for prolonged pain relief, often through a continuous lumbar plexus block. This technique involves inserting a catheter into the psoas muscle, providing extended analgesia postoperatively, especially after major hip surgeries [42].

6.4.6.2 Sono Anatomy

The ultrasound-guided lumbar plexus block involves targeting the lumbar plexus, which lies within the psoas major muscle near the L3-L4 vertebral level. Using a curvilinear ultrasound transducer, the key anatomical landmarks include the psoas major, quadratus lumborum, and lumbar vertebrae. The lumbar plexus, containing nerves like the femoral and obturator nerves, is located just deep to the psoas major. Care is required due to the proximity of sensitive structures such as the kidneys. Techniques like the Shamrock method is used for better visualization and safer needle placement (Fig. 6.7) [43].

6.4.6.3 Side Effects and Complications

Common side effects include local anesthetic toxicity, hematoma formation, and hypotension. More serious complications can involve nerve damage, accidental spread to the epidural or subarachnoid space, and infection, particularly with continuous catheter use. There is also a risk of injury to the kidneys or abdominal organs due to their proximity. Proper technique and careful patient selection are crucial to minimize these risks [42].

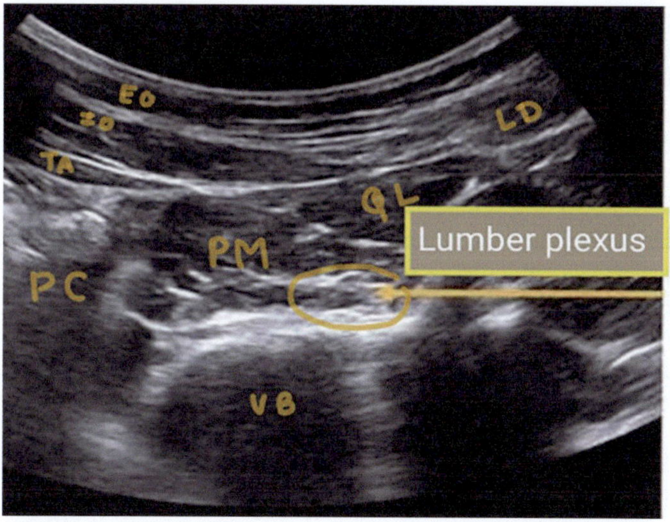

Fig. 6.7 Sono anatomy of lumbar plexus block at third Lumbar vertebral level. (EOM External Oblique Muscle; IOM Internal Oblique Muscle; TAM Transversus Abdominis Muscle; QL Quadratus Lumborum Muscle; ESP Erector Spinae Muscle; TP Transverse Process; L3 Body of 3rd Lumbar Vertebrae; PC Psoas compartment)

6.4.6.4 Femoral Nerve Block

The femoral nerve, the largest terminal branch of the lumbar plexus, arises from the posterior division of the ventral rami of the L2-L4 spinal nerves (Fig. 6.6). A femoral nerve block effectively anesthetizes the anterior upper leg and the medial portions of the lower leg. This block is commonly used for pain management or surgical anesthesia in procedures involving the upper leg, knee, femoral neck, femur fractures, and surgeries on the medial calf, ankle, or foot.

After emerging from the lumbar plexus, the femoral nerve travels downward in a groove between the psoas and iliacus muscles. At the level of the inguinal ligament, it is positioned approximately 1–2 cm lateral to the femoral artery. As it reaches the inguinal crease, the nerve remains lateral to the femoral artery but may shift closer, sometimes assuming a posterolateral position. Beyond this point, it divides into anterior (superficial) and posterior (deep) branches.

6.4.6.5 Sono Anatomy

A linear high-frequency transducer (15-5 MHz) is placed transversely over the anterior thigh at the inguinal crease to visualize the underlying structures. On ultrasound, the femoral artery appears lateral to the femoral vein, while the iliopsoas muscle is positioned lateral to the femoral artery. The fascia iliaca, covering the iliopsoas muscle, lies deep to both the femoral artery and vein. In contrast, the fascia lata is more superficial, positioned above the fascia iliaca and femoral vessels.

The femoral nerve appears as a hyperechoic (bright) structure lateral to the femoral artery, just beneath the fascia iliaca and resting on the iliopsoas muscle (Fig. 6.8). Using either an in-plane or out-of-plane approach, a short-beveled 22-gauge needle (5–10 cm) is inserted in a lateral-to-medial direction. The needle is advanced until its tip is positioned beneath the fascia iliaca and lateral to the

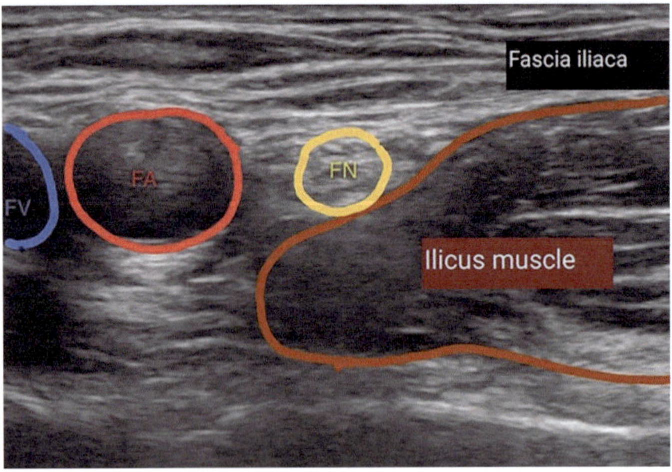

Fig. 6.8 Sono anatomy of femoral nerve block. (FN Femoral Nerve; FA Femoral Artery; FV Femoral Vein)

femoral nerve. After confirming negative aspiration, a small volume of local anesthetic is injected to hydrodissect and create a visible separation between the fascia iliaca and the femoral nerve. The ultrasound probe is then moved proximally and distally to verify the anesthetic's spread along the femoral nerve. A total of 10–20 mL of local anesthetic is administered in increments, with gentle aspiration between injections, while continuously monitoring the distribution of the anesthetic around the nerve.

6.4.6.6 Side Effects and Complications

The femoral nerve block is generally regarded as a safe procedure; however, it may cause motor blockade of the hip flexor and knee extensor muscles. This can increase the risk of falls, impede early participation in physical therapy, and potentially delay discharge. The risk of infection with a single-shot femoral nerve block is minimal, though it slightly increases when a catheter is used for continuous blockade [43].

6.4.6.7 Sciatic Nerve Block

The sciatic nerve block at the popliteal fossa, also referred to as the popliteo-sciatic or popliteal block, is a widely used technique. Blocking the sciatic nerve at this site provides a similar distribution of anesthesia as a more proximal block while preserving knee flexion, as the muscles of the thigh remain unaffected.

The sciatic nerve originates from the convergence of the ventral rami of the L4 to S3 spinal nerves along the posterior aspect of the ischium (Fig. 6.6). Each ventral ramus divides into dorsal and ventral branches, which correspond to the lateral and medial portions of the sciatic nerve, respectively. This lateral-medial organization is maintained along its course, with the lateral fibers eventually giving rise to the common peroneal nerve and the medial fibers forming the tibial nerve as the sciatic nerve divides in the distal thigh.

6.4.6.8 Sono Anatomy

A high-frequency linear ultrasound transducer is placed transversely at the popliteal crease to identify key structures. The popliteal artery is visualized, with the popliteal vein located just superficial to it, and the tibial nerve positioned just above both vessels. Due to the anisotropy of the nerve, the transducer is tilted slightly to enhance the brightness of the nerve on the ultrasound. The transducer is then moved proximally to locate the common peroneal nerve, which lies lateral and slightly superficial to the tibial nerve. Sliding the transducer further proximally reveals the bifurcation of the sciatic nerve. On ultrasound, the sciatic nerve appears as a round structure with a distinctive "honeycomb" pattern, characterized by hypoechoic nerve fascicles encased in a hyperechoic perineurium. It is most clearly visualized between the lateral muscle group (short and long heads of the biceps femoris) and the medial muscle group (semimembranosus and semitendinosus) [44].

Next, the transducer is moved distally to trace the sciatic nerve as it divides into the common peroneal nerve (laterally) and the tibial nerve (medially) (Fig. 6.9). Regardless of patient positioning—supine, prone, or lateral decubitus—a 20 to 22-gauge, 10 cm echogenic needle is inserted at the lateral edge of the transducer using an in-plane approach from lateral to medial. The block is targeted just distal to the sciatic nerve bifurcation, where the common peroneal and tibial nerves remain enclosed within a common sheath, separated by a narrow gap. Positioning the needle tip in the subparaneural space between these nerves helps avoid nerve fascicle penetration. This technique facilitates a faster onset of both motor and sensory blockade, ensures better longitudinal spread of the local anesthetic, and increases the likelihood of success with a single needle pass [45].

6.4.6.9 Side Effects and Complications

Although there are very few major problems from popliteal block, motor weakness is a major issue. Poor postoperative rehabilitation and patient falls might result from motor weakness brought on by popliteal block and other lower extremity blocks. The inability to dorsiflex the ankle, or foot drop, is the primary motor weakness linked to popliteal block. This results in the foot dragging and catching on the ground.

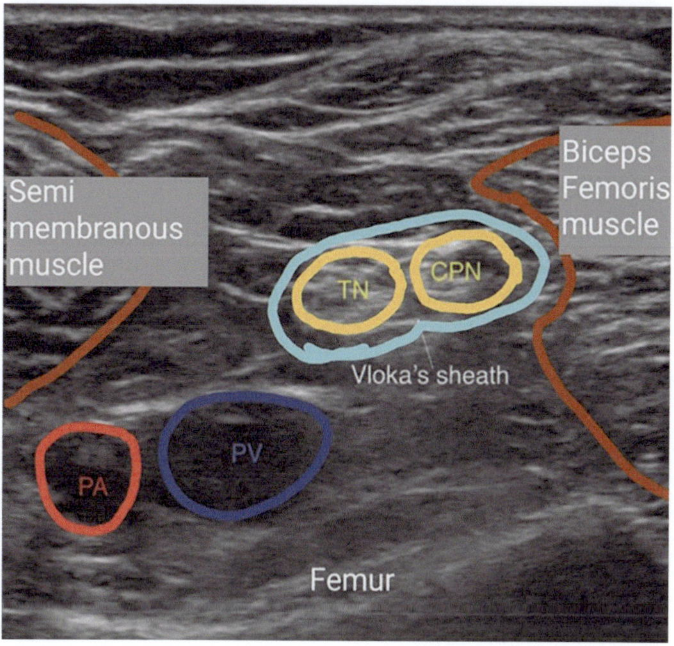

Fig. 6.9 Sono anatomy of sciatic nerve block at popliteal fossa. (TN Tibila Nerve; CPN Common Peroneal Nerve; PA Popliteal Artery; PV Popliteal Vein), Biceps femoris on lateral side

6.5 Conclusion

Patient autonomy in pain management is improved by patient-controlled analgesia as it allows for precise self-administration of analgesic medications. This improves both pain management and patient satisfaction. In a variety of clinical contexts, neuraxial analgesia continues to be a fundamental component of pain management. Technological and methodological developments keep improving its safety and effectiveness, offering useful alternatives for the treatment of both acute and chronic pain. For peripheral nerve blocks, a combination of careful technique, basic landmarks, and solid anatomy knowledge are essential for a constant success rate and lowering the risk of complications. These techniques will be further refined by ongoing research and clinical experience, improving patient results and pain alleviation.

References

1. Raja SN, Carr DB, Cohen M, et al. The revised IASP definition of pain: concepts, challenges, and compromises. Pain. 2020;161(9):1976–82. available at https://pubmed.ncbi.nlm.nih.gov/32694387/
2. Brennan F, Carr DB, Cousins M. Pain management: a fundamental human right. Anesth Analg. 2007;105(1):205–21.
3. Sinatra R. Causes and consequences of inadequate management of acute pain. Pain Med. 2010;11(12):1859–71.
4. Mann C, Ouro-Bang'na F, Eledjam JJ. Patient-controlled analgesia. Curr Drug Targets. 2005;6(7):815–9.
5. Aguirre J, Del Moral A, Cobo I, Borgeat A, Blumenthal S. The role of continuous peripheral nerve blocks. Anesthesiol Res Pract. 2012;2012:560879.
6. Viscusi ER, Reynolds L, Chung F, Atkinson LE, Khanna S. Patient-controlled transdermal fentanyl hydrochloride vs intravenous morphine pump for postoperative pain: a randomized controlled trial. JAMA. 2004;291(11):1333–41.
7. McNicol ED, Ferguson MC, Hudcova J. Patient controlled opioid analgesia versus non-patient controlled opioid analgesia for postoperative pain. Cochrane Database Syst Rev. 2015;2015(6):CD003348.
8. Hudcova J, McNicol E, Quah C, Lau J, Carr DB. Patient controlled intravenous opioid analgesia versus conventional opioid analgesia for postoperative pain control: a quantitative systematic review. Acute Pain. 2005;7:115–32.
9. Chumbley GM, Hall GM, Salmon P. Patient-controlled analgesia: an assessment by 200 patients. Anaesthesia. 1998;53:216–21.
10. Bainbridge D, Martin JE, Cheng DC. Patient-controlled versus nurse-controlled analgesia after cardiac surgery–a meta-analysis. Can J Anaesth. 2006;53(5):492–9.
11. Sellers CL. Avoid PCA by proxy. Nursing. 2015;45(10):9.
12. Grass JA. Patient-controlled analgesia. Anesth Analg. 2005;101:544–61.
13. Soffin EM, Liu SS. Benzon HT, Raja SN, Fishman SM, Liu SS, Steven P, editors. Chapter 13: Essentials of pain medicine. 4th ed. Elsevier Inc. p. 117–22.
14. Schug SA, Palmer GM, Scott DA, Alcock M, Halliwel R, Mott JF. Acute pain management: scientific evidence. 2020. Australian and New Zealand College of Anaesthetists. Available at: https://hdlhandlenet/11055/107 Last assessed Oct 2024.

15. Practice guidelines for obstetric anesthesia: an updated report by the American Society of Anesthesiologists Task Force on Obstetric Anesthesia and the Society for Obstetric Anesthesia and Perinatology. Anesthesiology. 2016;124:270–300.
16. Nishimori M, Ballantyne JC, Low JHS. Epidural pain relief versus systemic opioid-based pain relief for abdominal aortic surgery. Cochrane Database Syst Rev. 2006;3:CD00505.
17. Joshi GP, Bonnet F, Shah R, Wilkinson RC, Camu F, Fischer B, et al. A systematic review of randomized trials evaluating regional techniques for post thoracotomy analgesia. Anesth Analg. 2008;107:1026–40.
18. Svircevic V, Nierich AP, Moons KG, Diephuis JC, Ennema JJ, Brandon Bravo Bruinsma GJ, et al. Thoracic epidural anesthesia for cardiac surgery: a randomized trial. Anesthesiology. 2011;114:262–70.
19. Macfarlane AJR, Prasad GA, Chan VWS, Brull R. Does regional anaesthesia improve outcome after total hip arthroplasty? A systematic review. Br J Anaesth. 2009;103:335–45.
20. van Lier F, van der Geest PJ, Hoeks SE, van Gestel YR, Hol JW, Sin DD, et al. Epidural analgesia is associated with improved health outcomes of surgical patients with chronic obstructive pulmonary disease. Anesthesiology. 2011;115:315–21.
21. Ashken T, West S. Regional anaesthesia in patients at risk of bleeding. BJA Educ. 2021;21(3):84–94.
22. Macfarlane AJR, Hewson DW, Brull R. Spinal, epidural, and caudal anesthesia. In: Gropper MA, Eriksson LI, Fleisher LA, et al., editors. Miller's Anesthesia, vol. 41. 10th ed. Elsevier – Health Sciences Division; 2024. p. 1267–304.
23. Conlin N, Grant MC, Wu LC. Benzon HT, Raja SN, Fishman SM, Liu SS, Steven P, editors. Chapter 14: Essentials of pain medicine. 4th ed. Elsevier Inc. p. 123–8.
24. Hernandez GA, Grant MC, Wu CL. Benzon HT, Raja SN, Fishman SM, Liu SS, Steven P, editors. Chapter 15: Essentials of pain medicine. 4th ed. Elsevier Inc. p. 129–34.
25. Ngan Kee WD. Intrathecal pethidine: pharmacology and clinical applications. Anaesth Intensive Care. 1998;26:137–46.
26. Kurita GP, Sjøgren P, Klepstad P, Mercadante S. Interventional techniques to management of cancer-related pain: clinical and critical aspects. Cancers (Basel). 2019;11(4):443.
27. Smyth CE, Jarvis V, Poulin P. Brief review: neuraxial analgesia in refractory malignant pain. Can J Anesth. 2014;61:141–53.
28. Shatil B, Smiley R. Neuraxial analgesia for labour. BJA Educ. 2020;20(3):96–102.
29. Lin E, Choi J, Hadzic A. Peripheral nerve blocks for outpatient surgery: evidence-based indications. Curr Opin Anaesthesiol. 2013;26:467–74.
30. Ilfeld BM, Eisenach JC, Gabriel RA. Clinical effectiveness of liposomal bupivacaine administered by infiltration or peripheral nerve block to treat postoperative pain. Anesthesiology. 2021;134:283–344.

31. Johnson RL, Kopp SL, Kessler J, Gray AT. Peripheral Nerve block and ultrasound guidance for regional anaesthesia. In: Gropper MA, Eriksson LI, Fleisher LA, et al., editors. Miller's anesthesia, vol. 42. 10th ed. Elsevier – Health Sciences Division; 2024. p. 1305–30.
32. Kapral S, Greher M, Huber G, Willschke H, Kettner S, Kdolsky R. Ultrasonographic guidance improves the success rate of interscalene brachial plexus blockade. Reg Anesth Pain Med. 2008;33:253–8.
33. Vorobeichik L, Brull R, Bowry R, Laffey JG, Abdallah FW. Should continuous rather than single-injection interscalene block be routinely offered for major shoulder surgery? A meta-analysis of the analgesic and side-effects profiles. Br J Anaesth. 2018;120:679–92.
34. Franco CD, Williams JM. Ultrasound-guided interscalene block: reevaluation of the "stoplight" sign and clinical implications. Reg Anesth Pain Med. 2016;41:452–9.
35. Kessler J, Schafhalter-Zoppoth I, Gray AT. An ultrasound study of the phrenic nerve in the posterior cervical triangle: implications for the interscalene brachial plexus block. Reg Anesth Pain Med. 2008;33:545–55.
36. Sandhu NS, Capan LM. Ultrasound-guided infraclavicular brachial plexus block. Br J Anaesth. 2002;89:254–9.
37. Desgagnés MC, Lévesque S, Dion N, Nadeau MJ, Coté D, Brassard J, et al. A comparison of a single or triple injection technique for ultrasound-guided infraclavicular block: a prospective randomized controlled study. Anesth Analg. 2009;109:668–72.
38. Sala-Blanch X, Reina MA, Pangthipampai P, Karmakar MK. Anatomic basis for brachial plexus block at the Costoclavicular space: a cadaver anatomic study. Reg Anesth Pain Med. 2016;41:387–91.
39. Borgeat A, Ekatodramis G, Dumont C. An evaluation of the infraclavicular block via a modified approach of the raj technique. Anesth Analg. 2001;93:436–41.
40. Capdevila X, Bringuier S, Borgeat A. Infectious risk of continuous peripheral nerve blocks. Anesthesiology. 2009;110:182–8.
41. Gofeld M, Christakis M. Sonographically guided lumbar plexus block. J Ultrasound Med. 2013;32(8):1403–9.
42. Ilfeld BM, Ball SC, Gearen PF, Le LT, Mariano ER, Vandenborne K, et al. Ambulatory continuous posterior lumbar plexus nerve blocks after hip arthroplasty: a dual-center, randomized, triple-masked, Placebo-controlled Trial. Anesthesiology. 2008;109:491–501.
43. Morin AM, Kerwat KM, Klotz M, Niestolik R, Ruf VE, Wulf H, et al. Risk factors for bacterial catheter colonization in regional anaesthesia. BMC Anesthesiol. 2005;5:1.
44. Farag E, Mounir-Soliman L. Brown's atlas of regional Anaesthesia. Elsevier; 2017.
45. Leurcharusmee P, Yazer MS, Techasuk W, et al. A randomized comparison between single- and triple-injection Subparaneural popliteal sciatic nerve block. Reg Anesth Pain Med. 2015;40:315–20.

Perioperative Management of Opioid Dependent Patients

7

Ghansham Biyani and Nageswara Rao Tangirala

Abstract

The number of patients who are receiving long-term opioids has increased significantly over the last two decades. Perioperative management of such patients is often challenging and requires meticulous planning and multidisciplinary approach for successful outcome. It is important to take into account the psychological and physical dependence as well as associated comorbidities while anesthetizing these patients. It is equally essential to ensure that the baseline requirements of opioids are met independent of the anesthetic technique used. Use of regional blocks and non-opioid medications is found to reduce the opioid requirements and enhance recovery process. A small number of patients who are chronic opioid dependents and abusers may require very high doses of opioid medications in the immediate postoperative period for effective pain relief. Abrupt withdrawal of opioids in the perioperative period can result in withdrawal syndrome and hence must be avoided. This chapter delves

G. Biyani (✉) · N. R. Tangirala
Department of Anesthesiology, All India Institute of Medical Sciences (AIIMS), Mangalagiri, Andhra Pradesh, India

P. Ahluwalia (ed.), *Handbook of Perioperative Analgesia*,
https://doi.org/10.1007/978-981-96-7822-8_7

into opioid epidemic, opioid dependence, associated comorbidities, anesthetic challenges, and perioperative management of opioid dependent patients.

Keywords

Opioid dependence · Opioid tolerance · Opioid sparing analgesia · Non-opioid adjuvants · Regional anesthesia

Key Points

- Both opioid tolerance and opioid induced hyperalgesia are complex neurobiological phenomena involving multiple cell and tissue signaling pathways.
- Perioperative pain management of opioid dependent patients is often challenging.
- Two fundamental aspects of management in opioid dependent patients includes continuing baseline opioid requirements and maximizing the use of opioid sparing techniques.
- The use of regional anesthesia and non-opioid adjuvants as opioid sparing techniques must be considered in all patients to reduce the requirements of opioids and to provide effective pain relief.
- Multidisciplinary communication, planning, and execution are the keys to facilitate the best possible outcome in opioid dependent patients.

7.1 Introduction

The discovery of opioid medications is considered as an important milestone in the history of medical science, because they possess potent analgesic properties. However, the number of patients who are receiving long-term opioid therapy has increased significantly over the last two decades [1, 2]. This is primarily due to the large number of patients who are diagnosed with chronic pain conditions and malignancy are prescribed with increasing doses of opioid medications for providing effective pain relief. But, due to their significant addiction properties, a subset of patients develops either psychological or physical dependence and a few turn up being opioid abusers [3]. An increasing number of these patients are now presenting for various surgical procedures. Due to the underlying pathophysiology, opioid dependent patients pose unique challenges in their perioperative management [4, 5]. In this chapter we discuss the global burden of opioid dependence, various terminologies used, associated comorbidities, anesthetic challenges, and comprehensive management of opioid dependent patients.

7.2 Global Burden

- In the United States, the prescription of opioids has quadrupled in the last 15 years, leading to 1 out of every 5 patients with chronic nonmalignant pain taking opioid medications. The wide use of these drugs has led to an increase in the number of opioid abusers, estimated to be nearly two million at the end of 2020 [6]. According to Combating Drug Addiction commission, over 140 Americans are dying every day from opioid overdose [7]. As per the European Drug Report, in Europe in 2014, the average prevalence of high-risk opioid users among adults (aged 15–64 years) was estimated at 0.4%, the equivalent of 1.3 million [8, 9]. Similarly, an Australian study found that in 83% of patients with chronic pain and cancer pain, opioids were prescribed by the patients' general practitioners at the time of referral to a multidisciplinary pain center [10]. A national survey conducted in India on individuals aged between 10 and 75 years estimated that nearly 77 lakh people were addicted to opioid usage. About 10% of these were intravenous (IV) drug abusers with Heroin being the most commonly implicated drug. Majority of these abusers were from the states of Uttar Pradesh, Punjab, and Haryana [11].
- Most of the opioid enters into the Indian market either from the international network known as the "Golden Crescent" (Afghanistan, Pakistan, and Iran) or from the "Golden Triangle" (Myanmar, Laos, and Thailand).

- In India, opium poppy cultivation is prohibited under the Section 8 of the narcotic drugs and psychotropic substances (NDPS) Act 1985, except under a license issued by the Central Bureau of Narcotics under Rule 8 of the same act which permits legal cultivation in Madhya Pradesh, Uttar Pradesh, and Rajasthan only.

7.3 Definitions

The most common definitions used to define different opioid addiction status are briefed in Table 7.1 [1–5].

- *Opioid tolerance*: Tolerance to opioids is commonly seen in patients taking long-term opioid medications. Patients require increasing doses of opioids to achieve the same response, as prolonged exposure to opioids shifts the dose-response curve to the right. Hence, to provide adequate pain relief, either an increase in the opioid dosage or switching to another opioid is often required.
- *Opioid addiction (Psychological dependence)*: Opioid addiction is a chronic state, characterized by compulsive opioid seeking behavior and use, despite knowing its harmful consequences [4].
- *Opioid dependence (Physical dependence)*: Opioid dependence is a state of physical dependence, which occurs due to neuro-adaption to a specific opioid, characterized by the withdrawal crisis if the agonist administration is abruptly discontinued [4].
- *Opioid Induced Hyperalgesia (OIH)*: In contrast to opioid tolerance, OIH is a paradoxical phenomenon wherein patients treated with opioids demonstrate increased sensitivity to painful stimuli due to induced pronociceptive sensitization within the central nervous system. Patients may report hyperalgesia and allodynia, pain at sites distant from the site of insult, and widespread pain which does not respond to increase in the dose of opioids. In fact, treatment of OIH necessitates reduction in opioid dosage. The underlying neurobiological mecha-

Table 7.1 Definitions of opioid addiction

Opioid tolerance	A need for markedly increased amounts of opioids to achieve the desired effect Markedly diminished effect with continued use of the same amount of the opioid
Opioid withdrawal	The occurrence of characteristic withdrawal syndrome Opioid is taken to relieve or avoid withdrawal symptoms
Psychological dependence (addiction)	The opioid is often taken in larger amounts or over a longer period than was intended There is a persistent desire or unsuccessful efforts to cut down or control opioid use A great deal of time is spent in activities necessary to obtain the opioid, use the substance, or recover from its effects Important social, occupational, or recreational activities are given up or reduced because of opioid use The opioid use is continued despite knowledge of having a persistent or recurrent physical or psychological problem
Physical dependence	Along with the psychological dependence, there is evidence of opioid tolerance or withdrawal
Current use of opioid substance	It is defined as use of an opioid within the preceding 12 months (even once)
Harmful use of opioid	Current use of the opioid, along with scores on world health organization (WHO) alcohol, smoking, substance involvement screening test (ASSIST) between 4 and 26 (for alcohol, between 11 and 26), and experiencing any harmful consequence of opioid use within the last 3 months
Opioid Induced Hyperalgesia (OIH)	OIH is a paradoxical phenomenon wherein patients treated with opioids report increased sensitivity to painful stimuli and often necessitates reduction in opioid dosage

nism is complex and is likely to involve multiple cellular and molecular signaling pathways including glial cell activation, N-Methyl-D-Aspartate (NMDA) receptor activation, glutaminergic activation, and alterations in opioid intracellular signaling. To establish the diagnosis of OIH, apart from assessing habituation, tolerance, and threshold, the quantitative sensory testing (QST) has yielded positive results [12].

7.4 Anesthetic Challenges in an Opioid Dependent Patient

7.4.1 Preoperative

- *Difficult IV cannulation:* Opioid addicted patients are often difficult to cannulate as they inject themselves at multiple sites resulting in thrombosed and distorted veins. Skin abscesses when present also makes cannulation more difficult.
- *Capacity to consent:* If the patient is under the influence of opioid medications and presenting for an emergency surgery, taking valid informed consent becomes difficult.
- *Comorbidities:* Due to the chronic use of opioid medications, patients may develop various comorbidities affecting vital organs of the body (as mentioned below) and should be carefully looked into in the preoperative period:
  - Cardiovascular disease: Hypertension, dilated cardiomyopathy
  - Gastrointestinal disease: Reduced gastrointestinal motility resulting in increased risk of aspiration, dysphagia, constipation
  - Infectious disease: Hepatitis, human immunodeficiency virus infection, sexually transmitted diseases
  - Concomitant drug abuse: Alcohol, anxiolytics, benzodiazepines
  - Possible coexisting psychiatric disorders: Anxiety, depression, personality disorders

7.4.2 Intraoperative

- Patients are likely to be tolerant to the effects of opioids and may need very high dosage of opioid medications in the intraoperative period.
- Due to the lack of proven objective pain assessment tool, we need to rely on subjective parameters to assess the requirement of analgesia.

7.4.3 Postoperative

- Both underdosing (resulting in withdrawal) and overdosing (resulting in toxicity) are the concerns. It is important to watch out for withdrawal syndrome characterized by tachycardia, sweating, tremors, etc.
- Assessment of pain can also be challenging due to lack of specific pain scores. When assessing pain in individuals with opioid addiction, it is essential to consider biopsychosocial factors. The Pain Medication Questionnaire (PMQ) and the Screener and Opioid Assessment for Patients with Pain (SOAPP) score showed the strongest agreement [13].
- Opioid tolerant patients express higher resting and dynamic pain scores, and often require higher dosages of opioids. But the nursing staff may be unaccustomed to manage such patients and may be apprehensive in administering large doses of opioids due to the fear of causing respiratory depression and opioid toxicity.
- Patients with opioid abuse and dependence undergoing elective surgery have increased risk of postoperative morbidity and mortality, including surgical site infections, mental disorders, respiratory failure, pneumonia, need for mechanical ventilation, myocardial infarction, and gastrointestinal events.

7.5 Anesthetic Management of an Opioid-Dependent Patient

7.5.1 Preoperative

- As discussed above, both under and overtreatment is problematic in these patients. Therefore, an individualized and meticulous pain management plan must be formulated so as to prevent opioid withdrawal syndrome, provide effective analgesia, and to ensure continuity of care after discharge from the hospital.

- Formulate a plan for intraoperative use of opioid administration including the use of opioid sparing techniques (Multimodal analgesia).
- Continue oral opiates as normal: For elective surgery, patients should be instructed to take their usual dose of prescribed opioids on the morning of surgery.
- Convert requirement to oral and IV Morphine equivalents (Table 7.2). This is essential, as a subset of patients may not be able to take opioid medications orally in the immediate postoperative period either due to the nature of the surgery or for any other cause and warrants parenteral replacement. Equianalgesic tables are commonly used to calculate the equivalent dose of an alternative opioid (Table 7.3). However, a word of caution here, as the dosages are based on small studies, single doses, and in healthy opioid-naïve volunteers, they do not reflect the complex and heterogeneous clinical situations [1].
- Patches: The two most commonly used transdermal opioid patches are that of Fentanyl and Buprenorphine. Transdermal Fentanyl patch should ideally be maintained during the surgery. In case it is removed, a new patch can be applied in the intraoperative period. However, as it takes about 6–12 h to re-establish baseline analgesia, an IV infusion of Fentanyl should be initiated to maintain plasma concentrations. The infusion may then be gradually decreased in rate and eventually discontinued during this time period. Conversely, the efficacy of full opioid agonist like Morphine could be reduced

Table 7.2 Oral to parenteral equianalgesic doses of various opioids (in mg)

Drug	Parenteral	Oral
Morphine	1	3
Buprenorphine	0.3	0.4
Codeine	1	2
Hydromorphone	1.5	7.5
Oxycodone	1	2
Oxymorphone	1	10
Tramadol	1	1.2
Meperidine	1	3

Table 7.3 Oral equianalgesic doses of different opioids to Morphine (in mg)

Morphine 1 mg (Reference drug)	7–10 mg Codeine
	1 mg Hydrocodone
	0.5–0.7 mg Oxycodone
	0.25 mg Hydromorphone
	0.3 mg Oxymorphone
	5–7 mg Tramadol
	0.33 mg Methadone
	3.3 mg Tapentadol

by the presence of Buprenorphine patch. Therefore, if the acute pain episode is anticipated, Buprenorphine patch should be discontinued 72 h prior to surgery. Reconversion to Buprenorphine therapy can be done prior to or after discharge from the hospital. Another important concern about the use of transdermal patches in the perioperative period is related to the risk of altered absorption depending on the type of surgery, amount of fluids administered and body skin temperature, as all these factors alter the kinetics of drug absorption from the transdermal patch. Therefore, if a patient is coming for major surgery, it is preferable to remove the patch and administer equipotent doses of Morphine or other strong opioid agonists.

7.5.2 Intraoperative

- Intraoperative requirement of opioids should be guided by vital signs (heart rate, arterial blood pressure, degree of pupillary dilatation) and most recently by using objective monitoring like electro encephalogram (EEG) and analgesia nociception index monitoring if available.
- There is no data suggesting the superiority of use of any one specific opioid over the other. However, it is advisable to use IV opioid agonists having strong affinity to Mu opioid receptors such as Fentanyl, Sufentanil, and Morphine.

Table 7.4 Commonly used non-opioid adjuvants

Paracetamol
NSAIDs
NMDA receptor antagonists: Ketamine, $MgSO_4$
α—2 agonists: Clonidine, dexmedetomidine
Intravenous lidocaine
Steroids: Dexamethasone
Gabapentinoids: Gabapentin, pregabalin

Abbreviations: *NSAIDs* Non-steroidal Anti-Inflammatory Drugs, *NMDA* N-Methyl-D-Aspartate, MgSO Magnesium Sulphate

- Use of Remifentanil is controversial because of possible acute development of tolerance and hyperalgesia.
- It is very important to consider and maximize the usage of opioid sparing techniques: Multimodal pain management strategies using nonopioid medications (Table 7.4) and local/regional anesthetic techniques must be considered as part of the opioid sparing techniques in all the patients as it is shown to reduce the opioid requirements, minimizing opioid-related side effects, and risks of dependence [14, 15].
- A general outline of perioperative management of an opioid dependent patient posted for surgery under general and regional anesthesia is shown in Figs. 7.1 and 7.2 respectively.

7.5.3 Postoperative

- Patients warrant frequent bedside visits to know their comfort level and opioid requirements. This demands frequent alterations to their prescription and management plan.
- Multidisciplinary communication including pain services, physiotherapist, and psychologist is essential for optimizing the pain relief.
- It is advisable to admit such patients to either high dependency unit (HDU) or to intensive care unit (ICU) for the first 24 h following surgery so as to optimize their pain and opioid requirements.

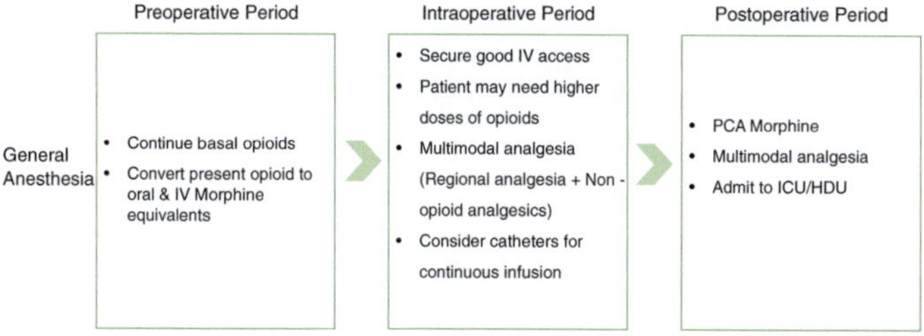

Fig. 7.1 General outline of perioperative management of an opioid dependant patient posted for surgery under general anesthesia. (Abbreviations: IV Intravenous; PCA Patient Controlled Analgesia; ICU Intensive Care Unit; HDU High Dependency Unit)

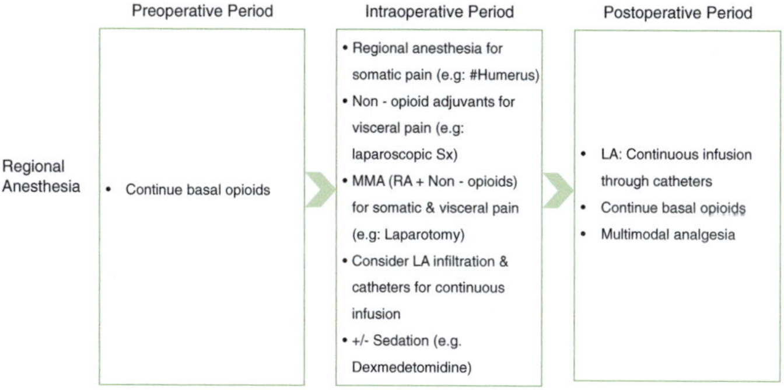

Fig. 7.2 General outline of perioperative management of an opioid dependant patient posted for surgery under regional anesthesia. (Abbreviations: Sx Surgery; MMA Multimodal Analgesia; RA Regional Anesthesia; LA Local Anesthetic)

- Opioid rotation: Switching from one opioid to another is a common practice in chronic-pain and cancer-pain management and is termed as opioid rotation. It is a useful option in those patients who have developed intolerable side effects or inadequate analgesia despite escalating the dose of opioid medications. Rotation can lead to both a reduction in side effects and an improvement in pain relief, because an individual may respond differently to an alternative opioid due to the phenomenon of incomplete cross-tolerance. When undertaking opioid rotation, it is recommended to reduce the calculated equianalgesic dose by 30–50% because of the possibility of incomplete cross-tolerance. Patients can subsequently use additional opioids as required [4].

- When assessing the overall effectiveness of pain relief, it is important to take many other factors into consideration. This includes the presence of opioid-related side effects, signs of opioid withdrawal, patient expectations and satisfaction, mood, and levels of physical function (e.g., ability to cough, deep breath, and engage in performing physiotherapy) [7].
- Use of patient-controlled analgesia (PCA) using Morphine is found to be a very useful modality as patients are made in-charge of their own pain control. They often require short lock-out intervals, running of a background infusion, and increased demand dosage for adequate pain relief. Two such examples of setting up a PCA for a patient dependent on either Morphine or any other opioid medications (e.g., Methadone) is shown in Figs. 7.3 and 7.4 respectively.
- It has been found that opioid dependent patients use 3–4 times more epidural Morphine and 4–5 times more IV Morphine for breakthrough pain relief in the immediate postoperative period to obtain good pain control. Moreover, the duration for which postoperative analgesia required in opioid dependent patients is about 3–4 times longer when compared to opioid-naïve patients.
- It is essential that one formulates and communicates a clear plan for onward care of the patient after discharge from the hospital.

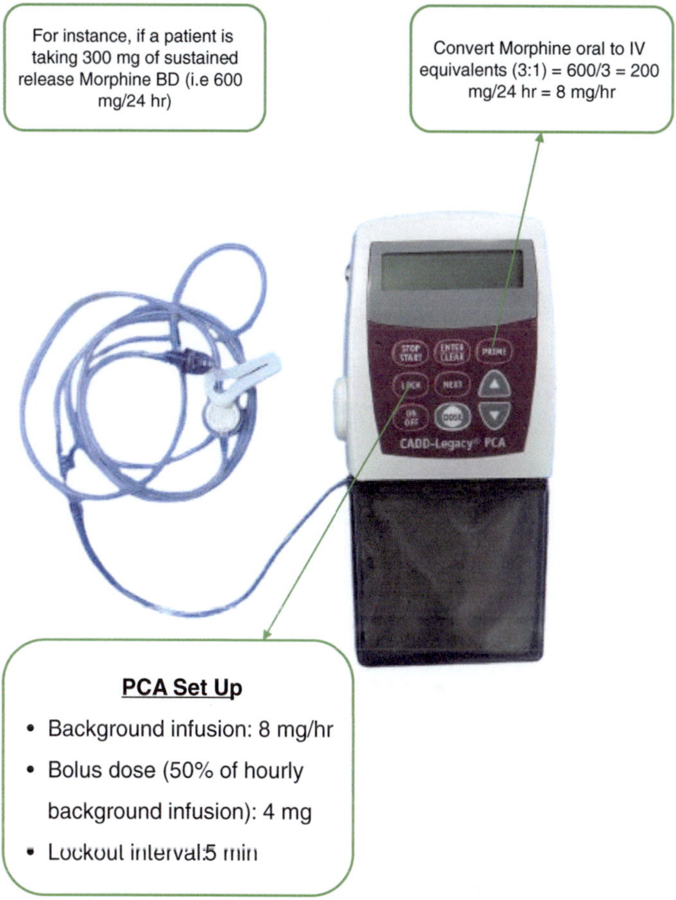

Fig. 7.3 Setting up a PCA in a patient dependent on Morphine. (Abbreviations: PCA Patient Controlled Analgesia; BD Bis in die; IV Intravenous)

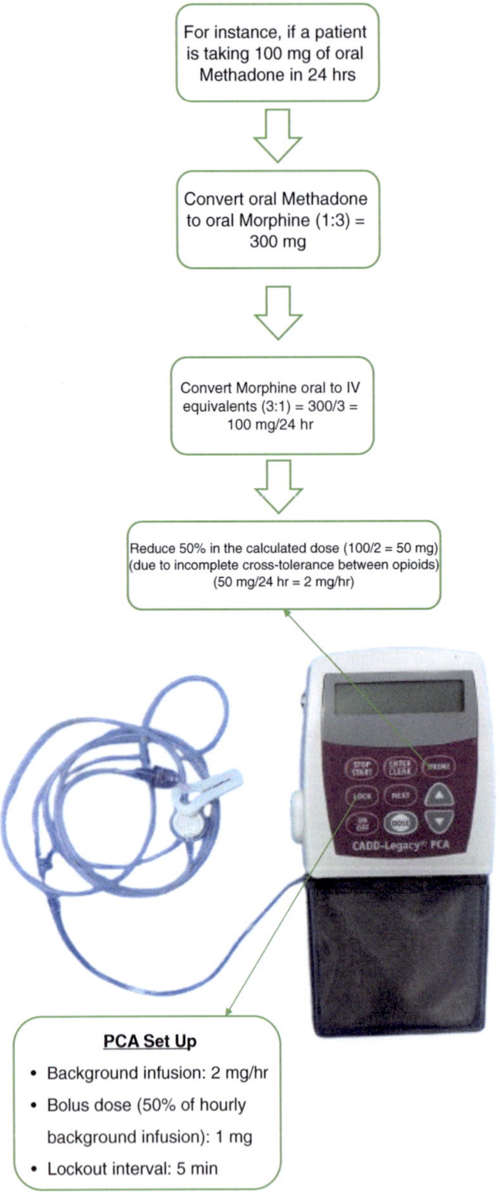

Fig. 7.4 Setting up a PCA in a patient dependent on another opioid (e.g., Methadone). (Abbreviations: PCA Patient Controlled Analgesia; IV Intravenous)

7.6 Drugs to Be Avoided

- Opioid antagonists, including Naloxone and Naltrexone, should be avoided in opioid dependent patients.
- Also, the use of mixed agonist-antagonist type of opioids which block the Mu receptors such as Nalbuphine, Butorphanol, and Pentazocine should be avoided as they could precipitate withdrawal symptoms.

7.7 Multimodal Analgesia

- Multimodal analgesia offers a comprehensive approach that reduces opioid use by incorporating a combination of medications and techniques targeting different pain pathways so as to achieve superior pain control with fewer side effects. By integrating the use of pharmacological agents and regional techniques, opioid sparing methods enables faster recovery and decreases healthcare cost [6, 16]. This topic is discussed at length in other chapters ("Multimodal Approach to Commonly Performed Surgeries" and "Drugs for Acute Pain Management").
- *Non-opioid adjuvants*: The commonly used pharmacological agents to reduce the opioid requirements are summarized in Table 7.4.
- *Paracetamol:* Paracetamol possesses moderate analgesic properties. According to 2022 multi society consensus, it should be used as a first line analgesic in the perioperative period unless contraindicated [17].
- *Non-steroidal Anti-Inflammatory Drugs (NSAIDs):* These drugs act by inhibiting the cyclooxygenase (COX) enzyme causing reduction in the synthesis of prostaglandins, thereby reducing inflammation and pain. These drugs should be used routinely to treat acute perioperative pain unless contraindicated.
- *NMDA receptor antagonists:* There is strong evidence to suggest that glutamate and NMDA receptors play critical role in

the development of opioid tolerance and increased pain sensitivity. Hence, treatment with NMDA receptor antagonists such as Ketamine and Magnesium Sulphate ($MgSO_4$) may attenuate the development of long-term tolerance to the analgesic effects of opiates. Ketamine at a bolus dose of 0.2–0.5 mg/kg, followed by an infusion of 0.1–0.5 mg/kg/h is found to be very effective [18, 19]. Similarly, there is data to suggest that $MgSO_4$ when used at a dose of 30–50 mg/kg IV bolus followed by 10–20 mg/kg/h infusion is associated with decreased pain scores and opioid requirements.

- *Alpha—2 agonists:* Both Clonidine and Dexmedetomidine provide effective α—adrenergic mediated analgesia. Clonidine at a dose of 1–2 μg/kg IV and Dexmedetomidine at 0.5–1 μg/kg IV bolus over 10 min followed by 0.3–0.7 μg/kg/h infusion are found to provide good analgesia.
- *IV Lidocaine:* Intravenous administration of Lidocaine is found to be particularly useful in abdominal surgeries like laparotomy by virtue of its analgesic, anti-inflammatory, and anti-hyperalgesic effects. The recommended dose is 1.5 mg/kg bolus followed by 1–2 mg/kg/h infusion for 24–48 h. A minimum infusion for 24 h has shown to produce moderate degree of analgesia, reduced opioid requirements, and improved bowel recovery [20].
- *Dexamethasone:* Steroids help in reducing the inflammation at the surgical site. Dexamethasone at 4–8 mg IV every eighth hourly can be administered in surgeries causing significant inflammatory reaction.
- *Gabapentinoids:* These drugs work primarily by modulating the voltage-gated calcium channels. Gabapentin at a dose of 300–600 mg per orally (PO) every eighth hourly and Pregabalin at 75–150 mg PO every 12th hourly are extensively used in the treatment of chronic neuropathic pain conditions [21].

7.7.1 Regional Anesthesia

- Regional anesthesia and analgesia are a cornerstone of multimodal analgesia, providing localized pain control by blocking nerve conduction from the surgical site.
- This technique significantly reduces the need of systemic opioids and enhances recovery. Other advantages include targeted and prolonged pain relief and decreased body's stress response to surgical stimulation. Hence, opioid dependent patients should be offered regional anesthesia or analgesia, particularly for procedures performed on the extremities [22, 23].
- Different regional techniques which can be performed include neuraxial blocks, peripheral nerve/plexus block, and local tissue infiltration. Insertion of perineural and fascial plane catheter to provide extended duration of analgesia should be strongly considered on case-to-case basis. This topic is discussed at length in another chapter ("Methods of Analgesia").

7.8 Future Directives

- The laws related to opioid cultivation and transport must be made most stringent.
- The prescription of opioid medications must be streamlined and tapering of the dose or stopping it altogether must be considered on case to case basis.
- Creating a centralized database system for individualized drug prescription and having a one pharmacy one user agreement in which a person can get the prescribed opioid medication only from the authorized pharmacy should help in strengthening the rules.
- There is an urgent need to validate a specific pain measurement scale so as to assess the severity of pain in opioid dependent patients as well as to maintain uniformity in data collection.

- There is also a need to conduct well-designed prospective randomized controlled trials focusing on the use of specific pain management strategies and their effect on pain relief and patient satisfaction. Moreover, studies should also focus on the long-term patient outcomes measured using quality of life and functionality.
- The future research should also be directed towards discovering an opioid having least addictive properties.

7.9 Conclusion

There is significant surge in the number of opioid dependent patients coming for various surgical procedures. Though we are now heading towards opioid-sparing strategies, the responsibility of providing a holistic care to opioid dependent patients is also bestowed upon us. As anesthesiologists, we use opioids on daily basis and hence play a centric role in looking after these subset of patients as we understand the unique underlying pathophysiology better. While anesthetizing these patients, one needs to address the associated comorbidities, note down the type and dose of opioid used on daily basis, and calculate the parenteral Morphine equivalents and formulate a patient centric management plan, as they all play a key role in successful outcome. Ensuring usual opioid intake on the day of surgery, use of multimodal analgesia, and prescribing Morphine PCA in the immediate postoperative period help in providing effective pain relief and improved patient satisfaction.

References

1. Veazie S, Mackey K, Peterson K, Bourne D. Managing acute pain in patients taking medication for opioid use disorder: a rapid review. J Gen Intern Med. 2020;35:945–53.
2. Mitra S, Sinatra RS, Warltier DC. Perioperative management of acute pain in the opioid-dependent patient. Anaesthesiology. 2004;101:212–27.

3. Vadeghani AT, Grant M, Forget P. Perioperative pain management interventions in opioid user patients: an overview of reviews. BMC Anesthesiol. 2024;24:310.
4. Simpson GK, Jackson M. Perioperative management of opioid-tolerant patients. BJA Educ. 2017;17:124–8.
5. Coluzzi F, Bifulco F, Cuomo A, Dauri M, Leonardi C, Melotti RM, et al. The challenge of perioperative pain management in opioid-tolerant patients. Ther Clin Risk Manag. 2017;13:1163–73.
6. Nicholas TA 4th, Robinson R. Multimodal analgesia in the era of the opioid epidemic. Surg Clin North Am. 2022;102:105–15.
7. Center for Disease Control. Prescription Opioid Overdose Data. Available from: https://www.cdc.gov/drugoverdose/data/overdose.html.
8. Allegri M, Fanelli G. Opioids and chronic pain. Data from the "other side of the pond". Minerva Anestesiol. 2017;83:6–8.
9. European Monitoring Centre for Drugs and Drug Addiction. European drug report 2016: trends and developments. Luxembourg: Publications Office of the European Union; 2016. Available from: www.emcdda.europa.eu/publications.
10. Nissen LM, Tett SE, Cranoud T, Williams B, Smith MT. Opioid analgesic prescribing: use of an audit of analgesic prescribing by general practitioners and the multidisciplinary pain center at Royal Brisbane Hospital. Br J Clin Pharmacol. 2001;52:693–8.
11. Ambekar A, Agrawal A, Rao R, Mishra AK, Khandelwal SK, Chadda RK. Magnitude of Substance Use in India 2019. Ministry of Social Justice and Empowerment, Government of India. Available from: https://online.fliphtml5.com/ljdmb/aacc/#p=1.
12. Lawrence R, Mogford D, Colvin L. Systematic review to determine which validated measurement tools can be used to assess risk of problematic analgesic use in patients with chronic pain. Br J Anaesth. 2017;119:1092–109.
13. Nunes JC, Costa GPA, Weleff J, Rogan M, Compton P, De Aquino JP. Assessing pain in persons with opioid use disorder: approaches, techniques, and special considerations. Br J Clin Pharmacol. 2024;90:2985.
14. Chen YK, Boden KA, Schreiber KL. The role of regional anaesthesia and multimodal analgesia in the prevention of chronic postoperative pain: a narrative review. Anaesthesia. 2021;76:8–17.
15. O'Neill A, Lirk P. Multimodal Analgesia. Anesthesiol Clin. 2022;40:455–68.
16. Ramaswamy S, Wilson J, Colvin L. Non-opioid-based adjuvant analgesia in perioperative care. Contin Educ Anaesth Crit Care Pain. 2013;13(5):152–7.
17. Freo U, Ruocco C, Valerio A, Scagnol I, Nisoli E. Paracetamol: a review of guideline recommendations. J Clin Med. 2021;10:3420.
18. Meyer-Frießem CH, Lipke E, Weibel S, Kranke P, Reichl S, Pogatzki-Zahn EM, et al. Perioperative ketamine for postoperative pain manage-

ment in patients with preoperative opioid intake: a systematic review and meta-analysis. J Clin Anesth. 2022;78:110652.
19. Schwenk ES, Viscusi ER, Buvanendran A, Hurley RW, Wasan AD, Narouze S, et al. Consensus guidelines on the use of intravenous ketamine infusions for acute pain management from the American society of Regional Anesthesia and Pain Medicine, the American Academy of Pain Medicine, and the American Society of Anesthesiologists. Reg Anesth Pain Med. 2018;43:456–66.
20. Eipe N, Gupta S, Penning J. Intravenous lidocaine for acute pain: an evidence-based clinical update. BJA Educ. 2016;16:292–8.
21. Davari M, Amani B, Amani B, Khanijahani A, Akbarzadeh A, Shabestan R. Pregabalin and gabapentin in neuropathic pain management after spinal cord injury: a systematic review and meta-analysis. Korean J Pain. 2020;33:3–12.
22. Leander M, Loon V, Lopez K, Ana M. Role of regional anesthesia in Enhanced Recovery After Surgery (ERAS) protocols. Curr Opin Anaesthesiol. 2021;34:616–25.
23. Memtsoudis SG, Poeran J, Zubizarreta N, Cozowicz C, Mörwald EE, Edward R. Association of multimodal pain management strategies with perioperative outcomes and resource utilization: a population-based study. Anesthesiology. 2018;128:891–902.

Acute Pain Management Services

8

Nitin Choudhary and Rohan Magoon

Abstract

Acute Pain Management Services (APMS), the concept dating back to the 1980s, has witnessed major developments over the last four decades. Initially, APMS was centred around the management of postoperative pain in patients with pain catheters or patient-controlled analgesia. However, in the present era, APMS caters to a wide array of patients which not only include the inpatient postsurgical patient subset but also those with acute or acute on chronic medical conditions such as pancreatitis and post-hospital discharge patients who still require pain relief. APMS comprises a multidisciplinary team that works together to manage various aspects of pain while aiming for improved patient outcomes. Various models of APMS have been described considering the limitations concerning manpower, finances, and infrastructure wherein every institution formulates a team best suited to its organizational structure and design. Having said that, with the ever-compounding complexity of the patient pro-

N. Choudhary (✉)
Department of Anaesthesiology, Pain Medicine and Critical Care, All India Institute of Medical Sciences (AIIMS), New Delhi, Delhi, India

R. Magoon
Department of Anaesthesia, ABVIMS & Dr. RML Hospital, New Delhi, Delhi, India

P. Ahluwalia (ed.), *Handbook of Perioperative Analgesia*,
https://doi.org/10.1007/978-981-96-7822-8_8

file, there happens to be an ongoing transition from APMS to Transitional Pain Services (TPS) which is more patient-centric with his increasing involvement in the contextual decision-making. Nonetheless, it is only possible in the backdrop of a thorough preoperative evaluation and history taking, that enables TPS to identify patients who are particularly at high risk of Chronic Postsurgical Pain (CPSP). The former indeed aids in conforming pain protocols to the specific needs and requirements of a patient. Despite all the benefits of APMS, its' role in improved patient outcomes is not recognised by insurance companies which regulate the diagnosis-based reimbursement rather than outcome dependency. The role of APMS/TPS is not limited to pain scores but it has a special place in Enhanced Recovery After Surgery, where adequate pain management features as a key component for successful implementation. However, it remains to be said that while evaluating the role of APMS/TPS in patient outcomes, it is time we embrace advanced tools, ahead of limiting our focus on traditional pain scoring systems.

Keywords

Acute pain management services · Chronic postsurgical pain · Patient-centric · Perioperative period · Transitional pain services

Key Points

- Acute Pain Management Services (APMS) began in mid-1980s for attending to the analgesic requirements of high-risk patients undergoing major surgeries.
- In 1990s, the Royal College of Surgeons and the College of Anaesthetists recommended APMS to be a part of the academic curriculum in all major hospitals performing surgeries in the United Kingdom.
- APMS team is usually led by anaesthesiologists and other team members include surgeons, ward nurses, psychiatrists, psychologists, physiotherapists, and pharmacists.

- The APMS pathway include patient assessment, intervention (pain procedure performed), documentation (the procedure performed, drug administered, any procedure/ patient related side effects, follow-ups), patient education, and audits, backed by a critical evaluation.
- Now APMS is not limited to inpatient postoperative pain management but includes pain arising from acute and acute on chronic medical illnesses such as pancreatitis, sickle cell disease, and acute exacerbation of conditions like inflammatory bowel disease, etc.
- The goal of APMS is to eliminate or reduce pain significantly while ensuring minimal side effects from the drug or intervention performed on the patient.
- APMS can have different structural organization like European model, low-cost Sweden modeletc.
- APMS is now getting replaced by Transitional pain services (TPS) as the role has extended beyond acute postoperative pain management to pain management due to various acute and acute on chronic medical illnesses.
- APMS is patient centric and in the growing era of shared decision-making various approaches have been developed to aid patients in taking an active role in decision making. Some of these include 'Seek, Help, Assess, Reach and Evaluate'(SHARE); 'MAking Good decisions In Collaboration'(MAGIC); 'Benefits, Risks, Alternatives, and doing Nothing'(BRAN); 'the Multifocal APProach to sharing IN Shared-Decision Making' (MAPPIN'SDM), etc.

8.1 Introduction

Acute pain management services (APMS) constitute a team of dedicated healthcare personnel involved in the assessment, monitoring, and treatment of pain as well as the management of the side effects associated with pain medications on a 24-h basis [1].

APMS commenced in the mid-1980s and came up with the definitive idea that a dedicated team of health professionals is required for regular and timed assessment of patients with a predefined goal of ensuring adequate pain relief which included written protocols and continued education of the health care professional involved in the team [2–4]. In the early 1990s, the Royal College of Surgeons and the College of Anaesthetists worked in unison on postoperative pain management and recommended that APMS should be introduced as a part of the academic curriculum in all major hospitals that are performing surgeries in the United Kingdom [5]. Over a period of time, APMS began to project the need for its organizational structuring as a crucial step towards achieving better inpatient pain management rather than diverting the entire focus on better drugs and their techniques of administration to the patient [6, 7].

Anaesthesiologists are usually the lead physicians working together as a team with other medical and surgical disciplines in managing perioperative pain. Anaesthesiologists play a pivotal role in decision making on multiple aspects of pain management such as the modality of pain relief, choice of analgesics, management of analgesics or procedure-related adverse effects, and, most importantly concern regarding patient safety during the perioperative period [8]. The APMS pathway herein ought to include patient assessment, intervention (pain procedure performed), documentation (the procedure performed, drug administered, any procedure/patient related side effects, follow-ups), patient education, and audits, backed by a critical evaluation. APMS, however, is not just limited to inpatient postoperative pain management, rather it's a complex medical service involved in acute pain management in all inpatients following surgery, pain arising from acute and acute on chronic medical illnesses such as pancreatitis, sickle cell disease, and acute exacerbation of conditions like inflammatory bowel disease, etc. [9]. Therefore, the importance of refined understanding of the core concepts of APMS cannot be overemphasized given the multifaceted needs of pain management in the current times (Fig. 8.1).

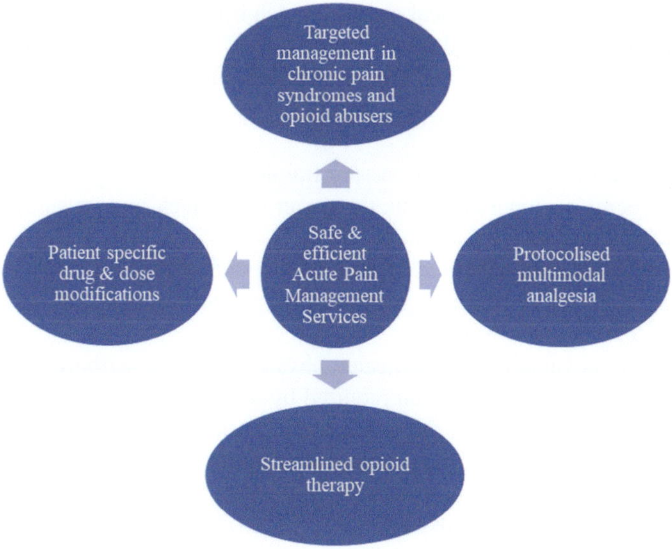

Fig. 8.1 An illustration highlighting the multifaceted attributes of APMS in the current scenario

8.2 Why Do We Need APMS?

Adequate management of acute postoperative pain is the fundamental right and therefore it is an essential component of a holistic approach towards patient management, in general. Pain relief ensures better patient outcomes with resultant early mobilization, reduced hospital costs, low opioid requirements, decreased length of hospital stay, and better patient satisfaction [10]. The goal of acute pain management is to eliminate or reduce pain significantly while ensuring minimal side effects from the drug or intervention performed on the patient [10]. Despite knowing the numerous benefits of appropriately addressed postsurgical pain, healthcare might not always be able to provide adequate pain relief to the majority of its patients. There happen to be various shortcomings in the healthcare sector which can potentially result in inadequate pain relief in postsurgical patients which is then at the root of the realization of the need for setting up APMS in the healthcare system. To cite, some of the major reasons for insufficient postoperative pain management, include [11]:

1. Physicians lack the necessary training in the management of acute postoperative pain, the newer techniques, and drugs, for that matter.
2. Shortage of experienced paramedical staff.
3. Lack of advanced equipment like patient control analgesia pumps in the hospitals.
4. Non-availability of dedicated physicians for prescribing pain medicines as and when required by the paramedical staff, i.e. non-availability during night and on holidays.
5. The nursing staff did not have the authority to dispense drugs.
6. Managing patients with catheters for pain relief requires additional manpower and expertise.
7. Lack of knowledge to the patients and their caretakers regarding the need for adequate pain relief.
8. Lack of sensitization by the hospital administration.
9. Surgical colleagues fail to appreciate the role of adequate pain control in improved patient outcomes and satisfaction.

The aforementioned reasons generated the need for the development of APMS to ensure pain relief for postsurgical patients. In 1988, Ready et al. [2] published an article wherein they proposed the concept of APMS to overcome these hindrances in better postoperative pain management. This new concept was a breakthrough in pain management which was exciting and was considered as a viable new opportunity. However, a fundamentally similar concept was also introduced parallelly at Kiel University Hospital and the US Command Hospital in the year 1985 [3, 12]. It was with time, that many institutions started APMS in their organizations tailored to their individual needs, resources, manpower, and financial support. Making local protocols that suit an organizational need can be especially helpful, in this regard.

8.3 Various Models for APMS

As discussed, APMS was initially started to foster postoperative pain services to patients undergoing major surgeries or to high-risk patients wherein pain management had a significant role in patient outcome. These patients either had an indwelling pain catheter like an epidural catheter or they were being managed with patient-controlled analgesia. Ready et al., in 1988, proposed that an APMS team should consist of multi-professional health-care professionals: surgeons, anaesthesiologists, ward nurses, psychiatrists, psychologists, physiotherapists, and pharmacists. This model requires a lot of manpower which adds to the financial burden and the complexity of functioning [2]. At the majority of healthcare institutions, formulating such an extensive team of multi-professional and multidisciplinary personnel remained unrealistic. Therefore, different models were developed to simplify the complex organizational structure such that more patients can benefit from using limited manpower.

Hence, there remains an inherent need for a successful APMS model to be simple and cost-effective. The APMS team should comprise highly motivated and enthusiastic healthcare personnel with diversely proficient skills [8]. Given these facts, a more simplified model i.e. the European model was suggested which consisted of a junior anaesthesiologist who was supervised by a senior anaesthesiologist [13, 14]. This model not only required less manpower but also provided a unique opportunity for the training residents wherein they get to be posted under the APMS team and learn the practical tips and tricks of postoperative pain management [2, 13].

Another model called the low-cost model was first introduced in Orebro, Sweden in 1991, which emphasized considering a specialist nurse as the principal workforce, to be supervised by a trained experienced anaesthesiologist. The specialist nurse would address all patients of varying age groups (paediatric to geriatric patients), take ward rounds, and then address the issues to the senior anaesthesiologist. This system worked on following standard protocols for pain management which were jointly developed by the team comprising of anaesthesiologists, surgeons, and the ward nurse. The specialist nurse is expected to facilitate the implementation of pain policies (assessment, documentation), coordinate teaching programs for ward nurses, and discuss special cases or patients who could not be managed on the lines of standard guidelines or any complication that required urgent intervention by a senior physician [7].

Of special note, the development of an APMS team requires administrative as well as financial support from both the department and the institution. APMS must be individualized based on the available resources and manpower. The third dimension of reimbursement of these services by the insurance companies is again very debatable and these further add to the financial burden levied on the institutes for starting such services, not to undermine the scarcity of resources at hand. Therefore, in the current real-world scenario, such services, especially in the most appropriate model, are feasible to start and manage only in major hospitals and academic institutes [15].

8.4 Components of APMS

APMS is a multidisciplinary team with different roles assigned to different team members. APMS model may vary because of different healthcare systems, hospital infrastructure and size, surgical spectrum, and lastly financial constraints [13, 16]. Minimal standards and consensus on adequate staffing are the key to high-quality APMS [17]. High-quality APMS is the result of a dedicated team that utilizes the given resources optimally with close interdisciplinary collaboration with other disciplines [18]. However, it's important to know the various components of APMS so that the tasks can be efficiently assigned and reassigned to different team members depending on the model and the requirements of the individual setup. Table 8.1 outlines the components and the roles and responsibilities of an APMS team.

APMS are patient-centric services, therefore clear communication between the patient and physician in-charge plays pivotal role in successful delivery of these services. APMS have

Table 8.1 Elements of the APMS team: the roles and responsibilities [6]

Components	Roles and responsibilities
Manpower/staff	At least one physician be available 24 h, with dedicated responsibility for managing the patients Senior consultant for supervision and to address complex issues Specialist nursing officer trained in assessment, management, documentation, and communication Training anaesthetists based on the model of APMS followed at the institute may or may not be part of the team
Additional staff	Other medical specialties such as surgeons, psychiatrists, psychologists, physiotherapists, and pharmacists Developing new pain protocols after taking the team's input and a thorough discussion Implementation of pain protocols inwards by the nurses Achievement of the rehabilitation goals wherein adequate pain relief has a key role to play
Teaching-training	Teaching programs for the staff physicians, training residents, ward nurses, and other members of the APMS team Communication with patients to make them an active member of the team Teaching patients and their family members, hospital administrators, and health insurance carriers Learning about newer techniques and drugs available for pain management Learning new pain protocols and enforcement regimes Research (as applicable)
Quality assessment and feedback	Regular data collection and periodic audits to study the feedback on the existing pain protocols Quality check of equipment to avoid any mishap Addressing economic concerns and devising new policies which would be more cost-resource friendly Assessment of patient-related outcomes by using more comprehensive tools Analysing the advantages and disadvantages of various analgesic modalities to refine the existing pain strategies Updating the current protocols based on the newer evidences and feedbacks Proper documentation of patient assessment as well as consultation notes

specific roles and responsibilities towards the patients that should be carried out by the designated team for better patient outcomes. Table 8.2 describes the patient-targeted roles of the APMS team.

Table 8.2 APMS: The roles and actions towards patients [6]

Role and responsibility towards patient	Actions required
Preoperative patient education	Provide comprehensive information regarding various pain management techniques with their associated side effects Counsel the patient regarding the expected outcomes from various pain management modalities Educate the patient about various methods of pain assessment Apprise patients regarding their role in decision making
Postoperative pain assessment	APS rounds should be twice a day Pain scores should be charted at timed intervals Side-effects or adverse events should be documented and reported Pain-related interference in daily activities should be addressed and managed accordingly Analgesic requirement should be individualised taking into account the functional outcomes Assess failed technique of pain management in terms of probable causes, and trouble-shooting techniques
Treatment adaptation	Consider patient needs and preferences before deciding pain management protocol Discuss and involve the patient in planning execution of pain management protocol Modify the existing treatment plan based on individual patient requirements Reevaluate the modifications in the existing treatment plan and its impact on patient outcomes Involve other medical specialties in inpatient pain treatment
Check out	Stop or deescalate the opioids on time based on patient assessment

8.5 Benefits of APMS

APMS was initiated to improve patient outcomes undergoing surgery with better patient satisfaction. Therefore, routine audits and analysis of the patient's feedback are important for refining the services to make them more suitable for the majority of patients. Some studies have shown that APMS was successful in decreasing pain scores with reduced incidence of opioid-related side effects [17, 18]. APMS with a trained professional team was able to quickly formulate patient-specific treatment guidelines for pain management [19]. It becomes difficult to study the role of APMS in decreasing the length of hospital stay, morbidity, mortality, and health expenditure, and ensuring patient satisfaction, as these are multifactorial [17]. APMS has been shown to decrease the postoperative opioid requirement by >50%, with early mobilization and oral feeding [18]. APMS has allowed the management of complex analgesic techniques such as thoracic epidural catheters which were previously managed in intensive care units to be now managed in wards. This has allowed a greater number of patients to benefit from such sophisticated analgesia techniques which was previously limited to very small number of patients. APMS has decreased the incidence of drug-related side effects such as nausea, vomiting, dizziness, and itching. Psychological components of postsurgical pain like pain-related anxiety, pain-related fear, and pain-related helplessness were less in patients managed by APMS. Patients managed by APMS experience lower pain scores and when required the APMS team acted immediately to ensure adequate analgesia for breakthrough pain [20]. However, it is important to emphasize that the mere existence of APMS does not ensure these benefits, it is team dynamics between the various disciplines along with a multimodal approach to pain management including regional anaesthesia techniques, opioids and non-opioid analgesics, co-analgesics, and other non-pharmacological techniques which ensures faster recovery with better patient outcomes [6].

8.6 Role of Shared Decision Making in APMS

The approach towards patient management has witnessed a great change over the past decades. In the present times, patients are epicentre of any decision-making pertaining to one's health condition [21]. This concept was proposed by Cathy Charles in 1997 and since then there has been a paradigm shift wherein patients are educated about the health conditions so that they can exercise the right to autonomy and be a part of the shared decision making (SDM) [22]. The present guidelines on APMS do not give clear directives on how to involve patients in SDM though they do emphasise on making it a patient-centric service wherein patients' needs, experience, and expectations are always taken into consideration [23].

There is growing evidence on the role of SDM in APMS and various structured approaches have been developed for this purpose such as 'Seek, Help, Assess, Reach and Evaluate'(SHARE); 'MAking Good decisions In Collaboration'(MAGIC); 'Benefits, Risks, Alternatives, and doing Nothing'(BRAN); 'the Multifocal APProach to sharing IN Shared-Decision Making' (MAPPIN'SDM), etc. These decision-making aids help in better involvement of patients in taking a shared decision along with physicians by overcoming organizational barriers and distant decision-making (post hospital discharge) [24].

8.7 Era of Perioperative and Transitional Pain Services

In the present context, APMS is not limited to the traditional management of acute postsurgical pain. It now encompasses a wide spectrum of medical conditions including inpatients with comorbidities requiring intervention for adequate pain relief such as sickle cell disease, pancreatitis, etc. [25]. The concept of APMS originated with the idea of postoperative pain management. But in the present era, this concept has evolved and is now considered as perioperative pain management which begins by educating the patients regarding the need for pain relief, the modalities available with their benefits, and associated side effects. The patient is well educated here to be involved in the decision making which allows for greater patient satisfaction [9]. Preoperative assessment of patients allows for early identification of patients who are at high risk of developing severe acute, subacute as well as chronic post-surgical pain (CPSP). Patients with preexisting chronic pain syndrome, chronic opioid dependency, substance abuse, and physical and/or psychological comorbidity benefit from tailored pain management protocols using multimodal analgesia techniques and the involvement of other disciplines for better perioperative management [26]. Patients on substance abuse can be screened for compliance with prescribed medications, opioid withdrawal for decreasing the likelihood of hyperalgesia, and timed intervention by other disciplines like psychiatrists to aid in better pain management [27].

While APMS decreases the length of hospital stay, the APMS team must extend its services during the post-discharge period for a specific subset of patients who specifically require it. APMS expansion includes postoperative follow-up of patients on complicated pain management and those on prolonged opioid analgesia for prevention or treatment of CPSP [28]. The transition from APMS to Transitional Pain Service (TPS) allows continuity of care in the postoperative period by following the patient's post-discharge with analgesic requirements or those who are at risk for the development of CPSP [11].

8.8 Future Vision

TPS is the cornerstone of Perioperative Surgical Home (PSH). The American Society of Anaesthesiologists endorses the concept of PSH for providing a cost-effective healthcare system. PSH is a patient-centric, physician-directed, multidisciplinary team approach that guides patients during the entire perioperative period. The patient is educated and involved in decision-making from the preoperative period till 30 days post-surgery. Another important component that is of special concern is the fast-track component in pain management protocols. In the present era of Enhanced Recovery After Surgery (ERAS), adequate pain control plays a pivotal role in its successful implementation. Guidelines should also here focus on inculcating the drugs and techniques that aid in early discharge and pain is one major reason for prolonged hospital stay and readmissions in the healthcare sector. APMS must feature as an important component for the successful functioning of ERAS, as efficacious pain control is very important for early mobilization which subsequently results in early hospital discharge [29].

Sufficient pain control is the fundamental right of every human being. The idea behind APMS is not revenue generation, rather it aims at cost-saving [26]. APMS forms one of the pillars of major multimodal rehabilitation protocols by providing good analgesia, decreasing opioid consumption, and early return to daily activities. A surgery should not be considered successful solely on the surgical outcomes such as the absence of perioperative surgical complications. Patient patient-centric approach should be considered wherein factors such as early ambulation, early oral feeding, lack of surgical complications, patient satisfaction, early return to daily activities, and the impact on the quality of life should also be taken into account [26].

Although APMS has been there for almost 40 years, its role in the healthcare sector is still not validated as a service by the health insurance companies. The reimbursements are directed based on diagnosis and the patient outcomes are still not taken into account by insurance companies. The surgeons have appreciated the role of APMS in the rapid turnover of patients, with early discharge. However, to gain maximum benefit from such services it's important to work as a multidisciplinary team approach [30].

Now the time has come that APMS should be considered a strong and definitive part of any healthcare system. APMS should be structured with a multidisciplinary team approach and utilizing the best available resources in the given institution. Its role is not limited to pain management but it has a significant role in shaping surgical outcomes. APMS helps by managing the complex pathophysiological changes following surgery by designing more comprehensive management protocols using the help of more complex assessment tools and techniques [31]. The pain assessment has expanded beyond the pain scores and multiple parameters focussing on the overall patient outcome is the new dictum. It is time to finally define high quality in the setting of perioperative care.

8.9 Conclusion

With the advent of APMS, postsurgical pain management has taken a completely different outlook. The benefits of adequate pain relief on patient outcomes have proven time and again which not only helped in the growth but also allowed these services to get their due credit in improved patient outcomes. However, in today's time, APMS is not limited to the postoperative period but it has expanded its scope to perioperative management and its importance in patient-centric management protocols. TPS is an example of a comprehensive approach that takes into account the preoperative as well as the postoperative pain management which in some patients extends even in the post-discharge period. The challenge in the future will be to define and implement generally accepted standards for organizational structures (e.g. qualified personnel), validated and agreed-on measures of patient-reported outcome measures, and continuous quality control.

References

1. Jain PN, Bakshi SG, Thota RS. Acute pain services in India: a glimpse of the current scenario. J Anaesthesiol Clin Pharmacol. 2015;31:554–7.
2. Ready LB, Oden R, Chadwick HS, Benedetti C, Rooke GA, Caplan R, et al. Development of an anesthesiology-based postoperative pain management service. Anesthesiology. 1988;68:100–6.
3. Petrakis JK. Acute pain services in a community hospital. Clin J Pain. 1989;5:S34–41.
4. Kuusniemi K, Pöyhiä R. Present-day challenges and future solutions in postoperative pain management: results from PainForum 2014. J Pain Res. 2016;9:25–36.
5. Gould TH, Crosby DL, Harmer M, Lloyd SM, Lunn JN, Rees GA, Roberts DE, Webster JA. Policy for controlling pain after surgery: effect of sequential changes in management. BMJ. 1992;305:1187–93.

6. Rawal N. Current issues in postoperative pain management. Eur J Anaesthesiol. 2016;33:160–71.
7. Rawal N, Berggren L. Organization of acute pain services: a low-cost model. Pain. 1994;57:117–23.
8. Kishore K, Agarwal A, Gaur A. Acute pain service. Saudi J Anaesth. 2011;5:123–4.
9. Miclescu A, Butler S, Karlsten R. The changing face of acute pain services. Scand J Pain. 2017;16:204–10.
10. Garimella V, Cellini C. Postoperative pain control. Clin Colon Rectal Surg. 2013;26:191–6.
11. Stamer UM, Liguori GA, Rawal N. Thirty-five years of acute pain services: where do we go from here? Anesth Analg. 2020;131:650–6.
12. Maier C, Kibbel K, Mercker S, Wulf H. Postoperative pain therapy at general nursing stations. An analysis of eight years' experience at an anesthesiological acute pain service. Anaesthesist. 1994;43:385–97.
13. Stamer UM, Mpasios N, Stüber F, Maier C. A survey of acute pain services in Germany and a discussion of international survey data. Reg Anesth Pain Med. 2002;27:125–31.
14. Rawal N. Organization, function, and implementation of acute pain service. Anesthesiol Clin North Am. 2005;23:211–25.
15. Sun E, Dexter F, Macario A. Can an acute pain service be cost-effective? Anesth Analg. 2010;111:841–4.
16. Nasir D, Howard JE, Joshi GP, Hill GE. A survey of acute pain service structure and function in United States hospitals. Pain Res Treat. 2011;2011:934932.
17. Werner MU, Søholm L, Rotbøll-Nielsen P, Kehlet H. Does an acute pain service improve postoperative outcome? Anesth Analg. 2002;95:1361–72.
18. Said ET, Sztain JF, Abramson WB, Meineke MN, Furnish TJ, Schmidt UH, et al. A dedicated acute pain service is associated with reduced postoperative opioid requirements in patients undergoing cytoreductive surgery with hyperthermic intraperitoneal chemotherapy. Anesth Analg. 2018;127:1044–50.
19. Fletcher D, Fermanian C, Mardaye A, Aegerter P. Pain and Regional Anesthesia Committee of the French Anesthesia and Intensive Care Society (SFAR). A patient-based national survey on postoperative pain management in France reveals significant achievements and persistent challenges. Pain. 2008;137:441–51.
20. Lovasi O, Gaál P, Frank K, Lám J. Acute Pain Services and pain-related patient-reported outcomes in Hungarian hospitals. Perioper Med (Lond). 2024;13:18.
21. Mihalj M, Carrel T, Urman RD, Stueber F, Luedi MM. Recommendations for preoperative assessment and shared decision-making in cardiac surgery. Curr Anesthesiol Rep. 2020;10:185–95.

22. Charles C, Gafni A, Whelan T. Shared decision-making in the medical encounter: what does it mean? (or it takes at least two to tango). Soc Sci Med. 1997;44:681–92.
23. American Society of Anesthesiologists Task Force on Acute Pain Management. Practice guidelines for acute pain management in the perioperative setting: an updated report by the American Society of Anesthesiologists Task Force on Acute Pain Management. Anaesthesiology. 2012;116:248–73.
24. Bello CM, Mackert S, Harnik MA, Filipovic MG, Urman RD, Luedi MM. Shared decision-making in acute pain services. Curr Pain Headache Rep. 2023;27:193–202.
25. Schwenkglenks M, Gerbershagen HJ, Taylor RS, Pogatzki-Zahn E, Komann M, Rothaug J, et al. Correlates of satisfaction with pain treatment in the acute postoperative period: results from the international PAIN OUT registry. Pain. 2014;155:1401–11.
26. Zaccagnino MP, Bader AM, Sang CN, Correll DJ. The perioperative surgical home: a new role for the acute pain service. Anesth Analg. 2017;125:1394–402.
27. Soffin EM, Waldman SA, Stack RJ, Liguori GA. An evidence-based approach to the prescription opioid epidemic in orthopedic surgery. Anesth Analg. 2017;125:1704–13.
28. De Kock M. Expanding our horizons: transition of acute postoperative pain to persistent pain and establishment of chronic postsurgical pain services. Anesthesiology. 2009;111:461–3.
29. Cannesson M, Kain Z. Enhanced recovery after surgery versus perioperative surgical home: is it all in the name? Anesth Analg. 2014;118:901–2.
30. Tran DQ, Krodel DJ. Optimal organization of acute pain services: at the confluence of semantics, logistics, and economics. Anesth Analg. 2018;127:808–10.
31. Benzon HT, Mascha EJ, Wu CL. Studies on postoperative analgesic efficacy: focusing on the statistical methods and broadening outcome measures and measurement tools. Anesth Analg. 2017;125:726–8.

Genetic Polymorphism Involved in Pain Mechanism

9

Baby Pegu and Dalim Kumar Baidya

Abstract

Pain is ubiquitous and difficult to treat and similar approach to pain management in all patients may not be justified. With knowledge of Pharmacogenomics, clinicians can develop an individualized pain management strategy. The majority of genetic variation occurs at the level of enzymes involved in drug metabolism which leads to differences in pain perception and drug efficacy. Patient specific genome testing may offer a comprehensive and personalized treatment.

Keywords

Genetic polymorphism · Pain gene · Pharmacogenomics · Opioids

B. Pegu · D. K. Baidya (✉)
Department of Anesthesiology, Critical Care and Pain Medicine,
All India Institute of Medical Sciences (AIIMS),
Guwahati, Assam, India
e-mail: dalimbaidya@aiimsguwahati.ac.in

P. Ahluwalia (ed.), *Handbook of Perioperative Analgesia*,
https://doi.org/10.1007/978-981-96-7822-8_9

Key Points

1. Genetic polymorphism seems to impact pain sensitivity.
2. Majority of gene variation occur at the level of enzymes involved in drug metabolism.
3. Variations in individual pain threshold, opioid consumption, side effects of drugs can be explained and treated better with the knowledge of genetic polymorphism.
4. Knowledge of genetic polymorphism paves the way to precision medicine in the field of pain medicine.

9.1 Introduction

Pain not just leads to individual suffering, it adversely affects activity, and functioning of hospitals and ultimately increases overall healthcare resource consumption [1]. Underlying genetic polymorphism may explain about 20–95% of the variations in drug responses demonstrated by individuals [2]. One of the important challenges in delivering satisfactory analgesia is interindividual variability due to difference in genes responsible for pain reporting, susceptibility, and pain sensitivity [1]. Genetic polymorphism may be found in various pathways including dopaminergic, catecholaminergic, opioid metabolisms, and various inflammatory pathways. New analgesic drug research may target on identification of pain phenotypes associated with single gene defects [3, 4]. Knowledge of genetic influence on normal and pathological pain processing would improve the neurobiological understanding of pain perception in both acute and chronic pain [4]. Moreover, pharmacodynamic and pharmacokinetic disparities occur due to gene polymorphisms associated with receptors molecules, transporter and metabolizing enzymes [5].

9.2 Definitions

Below we have discussed a few common terminologies which are often used while describing the pain polymorphism and knowing these helps in better understanding of the pathophysiology involved in genetic mutation.

- *Pain gene*: A pain gene is a gene for which one or more polymorphisms affect the expression or the functioning of its protein product eventually leading to alteration of pain response [1].
- *Pharmacogenomics*: The study of how genes influence an individual person's response to a medication.
- *Phenotype:* Clinical characteristics of an individual with a particular genotype.
- *Polymorphism*: A variation in a gene, deoxyribonucleic acid sequence, or chromosome.

9.3 Role of Ion Channels in Pain Modulation

The human genome contains over 400 channel genes. Ion channels are located in primary sensory neuron and play a crucial role in pain processing. Calcium, sodium, transient receptor potential (TRP), PIEZO, and purinergic P2X3 channels are mainly involved in pathogenesis of pain and are regarded as major class of drug targets for pain modulation [6–8]. Recent studies have demonstrated that abnormal expression of voltage-dependent ion channels plays important role in central and peripheral sensitivity, as well as in neuroplastic changes in pain, and inhibition of these ion channels could inhibit central and peripheral sensitization to alleviate pain responses [9].

Any noxious stimuli like a tissue injury are perceived by voltage-gated ion channels and this leads to changes in the biophysical properties, density, and distribution of the ion channels [10]. The pattern of changes in the ion channels depends on various factors including (i) age, (ii) sex, (iii) type of injury (neuropathic or inflammatory), (iv) duration after injury (i.e., acute or chronic), and (v) site of injury (i.e., somatic or visceral). Pain perception is associated with an increase in inward current of sodium and calcium channels and/or a decrease in outward current of potassium channels [10].

Neuron excitability after injury is perceived by ion channel, and as a result it affects the pain sensation. Sodium channels (Nav) have been the most widely distributed and most investigated and so far, nine such channel subtypes have been identified. Among them, Nav1.3, Nav1.7, Nav1.8, and Nav1.9 are primarily found in sensory nerves [1].

Alteration in N-type voltage-gated calcium channel (VGCC) contributes significantly to the transmission of pain signals in dorsal root ganglion (DRG). VGCC controls neurotransmitter release at nociceptive nerve fibers and modulates synaptic plasticity at the first synapse of the nociceptive pathways. In response to a noxious stimulation or nerve injury, VGCC opens, resulting in Ca2+ influx which activates protein kinase, resulting in development of pain. Calcium channel modulators inhibit Ca2+ influx and thereby reducing the abnormal excitation of pain transduction pathways to achieve pain relief [9].

The P2X3 channels which belong to the ligand-gated ion channel family are also important in pain processing. There are seven receptor subtypes named P2X1-P2X7 and are activated by extracellular ATP [8].

9.3.1 Acid Sensing Ion Channels (ASICs)

Injury and inflammation are associated with tissue acidosis and is a significant cause of pain. ASICs are activated during inflammation and acidosis (extracellular $pH < 6$). ASIC3 is most common type available in humans and probably has an important role in hyperalgesia and allodynia in inflammatory conditions [8].

9.4 Pain Polymorphism and Opioids

Opioids are the most widely used analgesic. Gene polymorphism may lead to wide variations in individual sensitivity to opioids and thereby clinical adverse effects. Pharmacokinetic and pharmacodynamic effects of opioids can be directly modulated by human genetic variations and polymorphisms of drug transporters molecules, enzymes involved in drug metabolism or opioid receptors. The human μ opioid peptide receptor molecule (OPRM1) gene has more than 100 polymorphisms. CYP2D6 gene polymorphism is the most significant polymorphism affecting opioid therapy. Others include A118G polymorphism, functional SNP (rs563649) located within OPRM1 isoform (MOR-1K). OPRM1 affects opiate sensitivity, tolerance, and dependence [11]. Figure 9.1 shows the correlation of different pain condition, their treatment modalities and gene polymorphism associated with them. The commonly reported genetic mutations and their effect on metabolism of commonly used analgesic medications is discussed below.

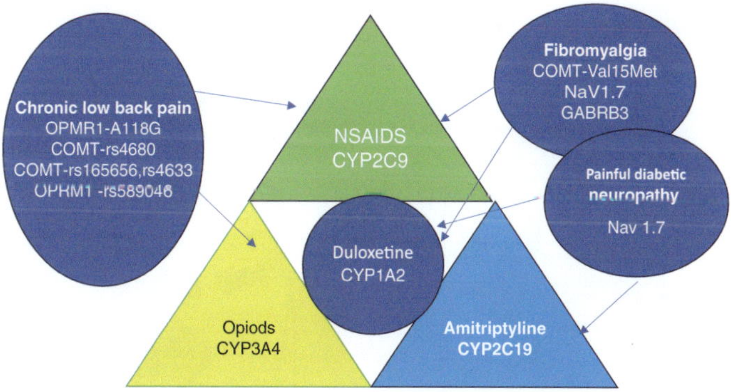

Fig. 9.1 Correlation of different pain conditions and their treatment with gene polymorphism

9.5 CYP450 2D6 Genotyping

Knowledge of patient's CYP2D6 phenotype can help physician in selecting most appropriate medication and decide on dose adjustment, thereby reducing its side effects. The CYP2D6 enzyme is responsible for metabolism of approximately 25% of drugs and demonstrates unique genetic polymorphisms that affect drug metabolism [2].

Codeine exerts its analgesic property occurs via conversion to Morphine and Morphine-6-glucoronide by CYP2D6. Poor metabolizer of CYP2D6 phenotype will have lower plasma Morphine levels, thereby achieving lesser analgesia compared to those who are rapid metabolizer (Fig. 9.2). Tramadol is also metabolized via CYP2D6 to O-desmethyltramadol which provides analgesia and hence poor metabolizer of CYP2D6 may tend to exhibit inadequate analgesic effects from Tramadol [5].

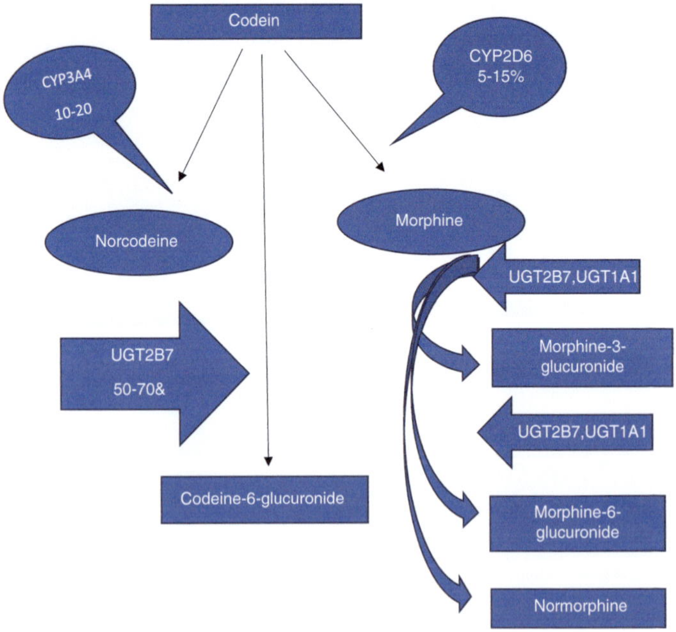

Fig. 9.2 Pathway of codeine metabolism

9.5.1 CYP3A4 and Fentanyl

CYP3A4 polymorphisms is related to analgesic efficacy of Fentanyl. MDR1/CYP3A4/OPRM1 gene polymorphisms may influence Fentanyl consumption and thereby affect its analgesic property [5].

9.5.2 UGT2B7 and Fentanyl

Uridine diphosphate-glucuronyltransferase-2B7 (UGT2B7) which is an Isozyme of UDP-glucuronosyltransferases, is involved in the metabolism of Fentanyl and the polymorphism of this gene may alter the pharmacokinetics and thereby clinical effects of Fentanyl [5].

9.5.3 ABCB1 and Fentanyl

Fentanyl is also a possible substrate of P-glycoprotein which is encoded by adenosine triphosphate binding cassette subfamily B member 1 (ABCB1). Genetic polymorphisms in ABCB1 may affect Fentanyl metabolism. A single-nucleotide polymorphisms in ABCB1 was found to be associated with respiratory depressant effect of Fentanyl [5].

9.6 Serotonin and Norepinephrine Reuptake Inhibitors

Duloxetine and Venlafaxine are serotonin and norepinephrine reuptake inhibitors (SNRIs). These drugs are used in the management of neuropathic pain, migraine prophylaxis, major depressive disorder, and in generalized anxiety disorder [2, 12]. Duloxetine has been approved by FDA for use in pain conditions such as neuropathic pain and fibromyalgia. Duloxetine increases the activity of noradrenaline and serotonin in the dorsal horn neurons of the descending spinal tract [12]. Duloxetine is metabolized to multiple inactive metabolites by CYP1A2 and CYP2D6 and hence it acts as a substrate and inhibitor of CYP2D6. Hence, CYP2D6 polymorphisms may alter its pharmacokinetics, pharmacodynamic, efficacy, and safety profile.

Venlafaxine undergoes first pass hepatic metabolism by CYP2D6 and gets converted to an active metabolite O-desmethylvenlafaxine (ODV). This is further metabolized by CYP2C19, CYP2D6, and CYP3A4 into other metabolites which have minimal pharmacological activity. Another minor metabolite of Venlafaxine is N-desmethyl venlafaxine (NDV), with weak serotonin and norepinephrine reuptake properties which involves CYP219 and CYP3A4 gene. CYP2D6 polymorphism results in elevated plasma levels of Venlafaxine [2].

9.7 Paracetamol and Pain Modulation

Paracetamol metabolism involves a number of enzymes and receptors. Cytochrome P450 monooxygenase (CYP) sulfotransferase (SULT), and UDP glucuronosyltransferase (UGT), and the receptors/ion channels transient receptor potential vanilloid 1 receptor (TRPV1), and calcium channels are the main receptors involved in paracetamol metabolism and its analgesic property. TRPV1 receptor has been shown to be a predominantly involved in paracetamol antinociception effect and its polymorphism is known to affect pain perception Similarly, a combination of UGT2B15 rs_1902023, TRPV1 rs_224534, and SULT1A1_rs_9282861, has shown to be associated with variations in paracetamol analgesic response.

9.8 Nonsteroidal Anti-inflammatory Drugs

CYP2C9, CYP1A2, and CYP3A4 are mainly involved in the biotransformation of NSAIDs and are subsequently eliminated by renal pathway. However, CYP2C9 has been found to have significant polymorphism leading to increased drug exposure due to hindering of metabolism to inactive metabolites thus exposed to more adverse effect of NSAIDs [2].

9.9 Genetic Polymorphism and Local Anesthetics

Clinical actions of local anaesthetics (LA) are correlated with mutations of the sodium channel genes [13]. Patients with chronic opioid intake have been found to have cross tolerance to local anesthetics due to an inhibitory effect of opioids on central and peripheral VGSCs [14].

SCN9A gene mutation demonstrates an increased resistance to lidocaine. In humans, amide and ester LAs undergo metabolism via different metabolic pathways. CYP3A4 is the main isoenzyme involved in the metabolism of lidocaine and bupivacaine whereas CYP1A2 isoenzyme in case of ropivacaine. Most esters are excreted renally after they are metabolized in to inactive compounds by plasma esterase. On the other hand, amide LAs undergo phase 1 metabolism either by hydrolysis (amidases) or oxidation (CYP450 oxidase system) in the liver. CYP3A4 activity has been found to have 10- to 100-fold inter-individual differences. Similarly, MC1R mutation leads to increased sensitivity to thermal stimulus and reduces subcutaneous lidocaine efficacy [13]. A molecular mechanism of resistance to local anesthesia has been suggested in patients with Ehler danlos syndrome probable due to altered local anesthesia dispersion. Patients with chronic opioid intake have been found to have cross tolerance to local anesthetics due to an inhibitory effect of opioids on central and peripheral VGSCs [14].

9.10 Advances in Gene Therapy for Pain

Although pharmacogenomic-guided therapy for pain treatment is gaining attraction in clinical practice, there are significant limitations in its widespread implementation. Safe and effective pharmacotherapeutic plans can be adopted by utilizing pharmacogenomic data. Efficacy and safety of drugs depends on the difference in enzyme metabolism status of the individual. An individual can have poor, intermediate, normal, rapid, extensive, ultrarapid, or indeterminate metabolism phenotype [2] (Table 9.1). The relationship between gene mutations, metabolism status, and variability in drug responses should be further explored. Therapies provided on the basis of genetic polymorphisms may improve the outcome of treatments and reduces the risk of drug-related adverse effects. Genetic testing of COMT haplotypes can help to predict level of pain perception and may be included in clinical practices. Thus, genetic testing for pain perception and drug metabolizer polymorphism would potentially be useful in clinical decision-making.

There are discrepancies in pain intensity scores given by patients and recorded by caregivers due to absent in knowledge of gene polymorphism. Patient's perspective of pain and suffering should always be respected [15]. Identifying the background genetic polymorphism may provide better understanding of relationships between pain development, intensity, and their response to medication identify new genetic targets for treatment. Moreover, better preventive and therapeutic pain management may decrease the overall healthcare service resource utilization and expenditure.

Table 9.1 Types of enzymic metabolizer with clinical implication

Phenotype	Genotype description	Implication
Poor metabolizer (PM)	No function allele	Enzymic activity is reduced, can result in treatment failure
Intermediate metabolizer (IM)	No functional allele or decreased functional allele	Reduced enzymic activity as compared to normal metabolizer
Normal metabolizer (NM)	Combination of normal function allele and decreased function alleles	Fully functional enzyme activity
Rapid metabolizer (RM)	Combination of normal functional allele with increased function	Increased enzyme activity
Ultrarapid metabolizer (UM)	Two or more functional alleles	Increased metabolic activity and can lead to drug toxicity.

9.11 Conclusion

The Human Genome Project Research has revolutionized healthcare by facilitating drug development and understanding heterogeneity in pain perception. Rapid progress in neurobiology, behavioral analysis, genetics cells, and molecular techniques have expanded the knowledge about the mechanism of pain transmission. Further advancement in research in the area of genetic polymorphism may provide better understanding of interindividual variations in pain response, opioid consumption, adverse effects, and complications and eventually may lead to development of precision medicine in acute and chronic pain management.

References

1. James S. Human pain and genetics: some basics. Br J Pain. 2013;7(4):171–8. https://doi.org/10.1177/2049463713506408. PMID: 26516521; PMCID: PMC4590159.
2. Brandl E, Halford Z, Clark MD, Herndon C. Pharmacogenomics in pain management: a review of relevant gene-drug associations and clinical considerations. Ann Pharmacother. 2021;55(12):1486–501. https://doi.org/10.1177/10600280211003875l.
3. Sexton JE, Cox JJ, Zhao J, Wood JN. The genetics of pain: implications for therapeutics. Annu Rev Pharmacol Toxicol. 2018;58:123–42. (Volume publication date January 2018) First published as a Review in Advance on October 02, 2017.
4. Carvalho Soares FF, Poluha RL, De la Torre CG, Costa YM, Nascimento GG, Rodrigues Conti PC, Bonjardim LR. Effect of genetic polymorphisms on pain sensitivity in the orofacial region: a systematic review. J Oral Facial Pain Headache. 2020;34(4):353–63. https://doi.org/10.11607/ofph.2641. PMID: 33290441.
5. Sun Y, Zhu H, Esmaeili E, Tang X, Wu Z. Mechanisms and implications in gene polymorphism mediated diverse responses to sedatives, analgesics and muscle relaxants. Korean J Anesthesiol. 2023;76(2):89–98. https://doi.org/10.4097/kja.22654. ISSN 2005–6419 • eISSN 2005–7563.
6. Zhang J, Yao J, Rong M. Editorial: role of ion channels in pain. Front Pharmacol. 2022;13:884665. https://doi.org/10.3389/fphar.2022.884665. PMID: 35734416; PMCID: PMC9207521.
7. De Loggu F, Geppetti P. Ion channel pharmacology for pain modulation. In: Barrett J, Page C, Michel M, editors. Concepts and principles of pharmacology, vol. 260. Cham: Springer; 2019. https://doi.org/10.1007/164_2019_336.

8. Gohar O. Contribution of ion channels in pain sensation in. 2005. www.alomone.com, pp 9–13.
9. Ma K, Cheng Z, Jiang H, Lin Z, Liu C, Liu X, Lu L, Lu Y, Tao W, Wang S, Yang X, Yi Q, Zhang X, Zhang Y, Liu Y. Expert consensus on Ion Channel drugs for chronic pain treatment in China. J Pain Res. 2024;17:953–63. https://doi.org/10.2147/JPR.S445171. PMID: 38476873; PMCID: PMC10929561.
10. Gold MS. Voltage-gated ion channels and pain. In: Binder MD, Hirokawa N, Windhorst U, editors. Encyclopedia of neuroscience. Berlin/Heidelberg: Springer; 2009. https://doi.org/10.1007/978-3-540-29678-2_6407.
11. Vieira CMP, Fragoso RM, Pereira D, Medeiros R. Pain polymorphisms and opioids: an evidence based review. Mol Med Rep. 2019; https://doi.org/10.3892/mmr.2018.9792.
12. Dhaliwal JS, Spurling BC, Molla M. Duloxetine. 2023 May 29. In: StatPearls [Internet]. Treasure Island (FL): StatPearls Publishing; 2024.
13. Cregg R, Russo G, Gubbay A, Branford R, Sato H. Pharmacogenetics of analgesic drugs. Br J Pain. 2013;7(4):189–208. https://doi.org/10.1177/2049463713507139. PMID: 26516523; PMCID: PMC4590162.
14. Marti F, et al. Resistance to local anaesthetics: a literature review. Br J Anaesthesia. 2022;129(2):e43–5. https://doi.org/10.1016/j.bja.2022.04.029.
15. Li S, van Boekel RLM, van den Heuvel SAS, Coenen MJH, Vissers KCP. Pain predict genetics: protocol for a prospective observational study of clinical and genetic factors to predict the development of postoperative pain. BMJ Open. 2022;12(11):e066134. https://doi.org/10.1136/bmjopen-2022-066134. PMID: 36446453; PMCID: PMC9710368.

Special Considerations of Perioperative Pain Management in Children

10

Kamna Kakkar and Bhavna Gupta

Abstract

Pain due to surgical and diagnostic procedures in infants and children is usually undiagnosed and undertreated due to lack of awareness among physicians and paucity of experience in treating it. This chapter touches upon the reasons and ethics behind the need to treat perioperative pediatric pain and includes relevant age-appropriate tools to assess it. Both non-pharmacological and pharmacological methods are being utilized to manage this pain. Use of newer modalities like ultrasound-guided regional blocks and non-opioid analgesics to prevent and reduce dependence upon opioids is also emphasized upon. A good perioperative protocol- to manage physical, emotional and psychological aspects of pain in children prevents long term complications like chronic pain, behavioral issues and mental disorders.

K. Kakkar
Department of Anaesthesiology, Faculty of Medical and Health Sciences, SGT University, Gurugram, Haryana, India
e-mail: kamnakakkar_fmhs@sgtuniversity.org

B. Gupta (✉)
Department of Anesthesiology, Critical Care and Pain, All India Institute of Medical Sciences (AIIMS), Rishikesh, Uttarakhand, India

P. Ahluwalia (ed.), *Handbook of Perioperative Analgesia*,
https://doi.org/10.1007/978-981-96-7822-8_10

Keywords

Pediatric Surgical Pain Management · Perioperative Pain in Children · Pediatric Anesthesia · Pediatric Regional Anesthesia

Key Points

- Pain is a subjective and unpleasant experience that affects children, especially during hospitalization due to surgical and diagnostic procedures.
- Effective pain management is essential for physical comfort and long-term mental and emotional well-being.
- Despite awareness among anesthesiologists and surgeons, a significant percentage (70%) of children experience moderate to severe pain post-surgery, indicating a critical need for improved management practices.
- Prolonged pain exposure in children can affect central nervous system (CNS) development, leading to altered pain sensitivity and increased risk of chronic pain syndromes in adulthood.
- Regular pain assessment is vital for effective analgesia and should consider various influencing factors (e.g., age, emotional state, prior experiences).
- Unique assessment tools like FLACC and CRIES are used for different age groups, along with scales like VAS and NRS for older children.
- Ultrasound can be employed to give basic and advanced nerve blocks for opioid sparing analgesia. Newer modalities employing Artificial intelligence are being developed for pain control in children.

10.1 Introduction

Pain is a subjective and unpleasant sensory and emotional experience, and acute pain can affect individuals of all ages, including children. In the pediatric population, painful diagnostic and surgical procedures are the primary causes of acute pain during hospitalization. Managing pain effectively in children is not only crucial for their physical comfort but also for their long term mental and emotional well-being. Additionally, ensuring an adequate level of analgesia, sedation, and nerve block at the surgical site is essential for maintaining homeostasis in pediatric surgical patients. Despite widespread awareness, studies show that 70% of children undergoing surgery experience moderate to severe pain, which highlights the need for improved pain management practices in this vulnerable population [1–3].

10.1.1 Challenges in Pediatric Pain Management

Several barriers contribute to ineffective pain management in pediatric patients. These include:

- *Lack of knowledge:* Many healthcare professionals are reluctant to use opioids or nerve blocks in children due to fear of adverse effects, and often leading to inadequate analgesia.
- *Lack of standardized pain-management protocols*: Due to absence of clear guidelines, policies or standardized pain management regimens children recieve an inconsistent care perioperatively.
- *Under estimating pain:* Some healthcare personnel may underestimate the pain children experience or prioritize other clinical tasks over pain management.

Hospitals that implement standardized pain management protocols and provide ongoing education on pediatric pain management demonstrate significantly better outcomes in terms of pain relief for children [4–6].

10.1.2 Consequences of Untreated Pain in Children

Consequences of untreated pain in children extend beyond immediate discomfort. The immature central nervous system (CNS) of children, particularly in the early years of life, makes effective pain management crucial for normal development. Maturation of CNS structures, including the myelination of nerve fibers, continues into adulthood, with peak activity during the first 2 years of life. Chronic pain exposure during this critical developmental period can adversely affect CNS development, leading to altered pain sensitivity later in life. Insufficient analgesia in neonates undergoing surgery or painful procedures has been linked to lower pain thresholds and chronic pain syndromes in adulthood. Prolonged or severe pain post-surgery, particularly lasting more than 2 weeks, increases the risk of chronic pain development within a year [7–10].

10.1.3 Ethical and Legal Aspects of Pain Management in Children

Effective pain management is not only a clinical necessity but also a fundamental human right. This principle was reiterated in the 13th World Congress on Pain (2010) in Montreal, which stated that children have the right to relief from suffering. In some countries, like Poland, legal provisions guarantee the right to relief and treatment of pain [11–14].

10.1.4 Safety Considerations in Pediatric Analgesia

The safety of pediatric analgesia hinges on preventing errors during the prescription, administration, and monitoring side-effects of pain medications. Preoperative education for healthcare professionals, children, and their parents is essential regarding understanding of analgesic drugs, their dosages as per weight, age, contraindications, and potential adverse effects. Clear communication with parents about the procedures and pain management expectations enhances outcomes. Proper record-keeping, including adherence to pain management protocols, regular pain assessments, and vigilant monitoring for adverse reactions, is imperative [14, 15].

10.1.5 Pediatric Pain Assessment Methods

Assessing pain in children is crucial to achieve effective analgesia and must be performed regularly. Pediatric pain, like in adults, is influenced by a variety of factors, including the surgical procedure, age, emotional state, anxiety, prior pain experiences, genetic predispositions, and environmental factors.

10.1.5.1 Pain Intensity Assessment in Neonates/Infants

Neonates and young children pose unique challenges, as they are unable to verbalize their discomfort. Observable signs such as agitation, crying, facial expressions, and changes in physiological parameters (e.g., tachycardia, elevated blood pressure) are often used as proxies for pain, although these signs may be influenced by non-pain-related factors (e.g., cold or hunger). Commonly used pain scoring systems in pediatric age group is discussed separately in another chapter on "Assessment of Acute Pain." Only a few are discussed here in brief (Table 10.1):

10.1.5.2 Pain Intensity Assessment in Older Pediatric Patients

1. *Self-Report Pain Scales*

For older children, self-report pain scales are effective tools for measuring pain intensity:

- *FACES Scale (Wong-Baker):* Suitable for children aged 3–18 years. It uses six drawings of faces with expressions that range from no pain (0 points) to the worst possible pain (10 points).
- *Faces Pain Scale - Revised:* For children aged 4–12 years. It features six faces, with scores assigned by the child ranging from 0 to 10 points.
- *VAS Scale (Visual Analogue Scale):* For children aged 3–18 years. This scale uses a 10 cm line, where 0 represents no pain and 10 represents the worst pain imaginable.

Table 10.1 Commonly used scales in pediatric pain management [26]

Scale	Parameters assessed	Outcome and scoring	Application
Premature Infant Pain Profile (PIPP)	Age from conception, behavior, pulse, hemoglobin oxygen saturation, raising of eyebrows, tightening of eyelids, nasolabial sulcus	Scored 0–21, with each parameter scored 0–3 points. Minimal pain ≤6, moderate-to-severe pain >12	Procedural and postoperative pain
FLACC (Face, Legs, Activity, Cry, Consolability)	Facial expression, leg position, activity, cry, consolability	Scored 0–10, with each parameter scored 0–2 points. Moderate pain >4, severe pain >7	Procedural and postoperative pain
COMFORT Scale (Behavioral and Physiological Parameters)	Wakefulness, mood, reaction to ventilator breathing, ambulation, muscle tone, facial expressions, mean arterial pressure (MAP), heart rate (HR)	Scored 8–40, with each parameter scored 1–5 points. Sufficient sedation 17–26, insufficient sedation/analgesia >27	Pain and sedation in neonatal intensive care units
CRIES (Crying, Requirement for Oxygen, Increased HR, Expression, Sleeplessness)	Crying, demand for additional oxygen supply to maintain saturation > 95%, heart rate, facial expressions, sleep patterns	Scored 0–10, with each parameter scored 0–2 points. Moderate pain >4, severe pain >7	Postoperative pain in neonatal intensive care units

Premature Infant Pain Profile (PIPP): Incorporates factors such as gestational age and oxygen saturation. It's useful for both procedural and postoperative pain, with higher scores indicating more severe pain
FLACC Scale: Measures five parameters (face, legs, activity, cry, and consolability) and is quick to administer for assessing procedural and postoperative pain
COMFORT Scale: Evaluates both behavioral and physiological aspects, making it effective in NICU settings for assessing pain and sedation levels
CRIES Scale: Specifically designed for postoperative pain in neonates, it takes into account crying, oxygen requirements, heart rate, facial expressions, and sleep disruptions

- *NRS Scale (Numeric Rating Scale):* Also suitable for children aged 3–18 years, this scale rates pain on a scale of 0–10, with 0 being no pain and 10 being the worst possible pain.
- *Pieces of Hurt Tool:* For children aged 3–18 years, which uses objects to represent the degree of pain experienced.

2. *Behavior-Based Pain Scales*

For children who cannot effectively communicate their pain, observational scales based on behavior and physiological parameters are commonly used: *FLACC Scale (Face, Legs, Activity, Cry, Consolability), PPPM Scale (Parents' Postoperative Pain Measure), and COMFORT Scale.*

10.1.5.3 Pain Scales for Children with Cognitive Impairment

For children with cognitive impairments, specialized scales are employed:

- *NCCPC-PV Scale (Non-Communicating Children's Pain Checklist—Postoperative Version):* Suitable for children aged 3–18 years.
- *PPP Scale (Pediatric Pain Profile):* Designed for children aged 1–18 years.
- *FLACC Scale-Revised:* Adjusted for children with cognitive impairments, aged 4–18 years.
- *INRS (Individualized Numeric Rating Scale):* Used for children aged 3–18 years with cognitive impairments.

Pain intensity is often categorized as:

- *Mild*: 1–3 points on the VAS/NRS/FLACC scales
- *Moderate*: 4–6 points
- *Severe:* 7 or more points

Pain intensity must be assessed both at rest and during movement (e.g., coughing, walking). Pain management should aim to reduce pain to levels tolerable for the patient, with a target of complete pain relief when possible [16–21].

10.1.6 Basic Principles of Pain Management in Children

Effective pain management in pediatric patients is crucial to improving recovery outcomes, particularly within perioperative care protocols, such as e*nhanced Recovery After Surgery (eRAS).* These protocols emphasize the importance of regular pain assessment (at least three times a day) and consistent documentation, much like monitoring vital signs. Below are the key principles of acute pain management in children, incorporating both pharmacological and non-pharmacological methods: [13–18]

- *Individualized Approach:* When selecting analgesia, factors like the child's age, previous pain experiences, type of surgery, expected pain intensity, and duration must be considered.
- *Scheduled Analgesia:* Analgesics should be administered at regular intervals based on age-related pharmacokinetics or via continuous infusions to maintain constant therapeutic blood levels and ensure effective pain control. On-demand dosing should be avoided; however, rescue doses should be available for breakthrough pain.
- *Pre-emptive Analgesia:* Pre-emptive analgesia is crucial for preventing severe postoperative pain and reducing the need for analgesics afterward. This involves administering analgesics before the onset of pain.
- *Multimodal Analgesia in Pediatric Pain Management:* This approach combines various drugs and techniques that target different mechanisms involved in pain transduction and perception. The combination of analgesics, co-analgesics, and regional/local anesthesia techniques is key to ensuring effective analgesia, thus optimizing perioperative pain management in pediatric patients [22–25].
- *Monitoring of Pain: Regular* monitoring of pain, at least three times daily, is essential. New devices aimed at improving pain

assessment in young children, particularly in ICUs, are under development. These devices often rely on heart rate variability or changes in the parasympathetic system to optimize pain management. Machine learning and Deep Learning, both subsets of the Artificial Intelligence spectrum, are being employed to develop programs to identify and treat pain in children, safely and effectively [26, 27].

- *Postoperative Considerations*
  - As per ERAS Society protocol for neonatal patients, in post-operative period, opioid use is to be limited but if in case, opioids are needed, lowest effective dose with continuous monitoring are recommended.
  - Paracetamol/Acetaminophen is recommended to be given regularly in the early post-operative period and not on a "as per need" basis along with continuation of multi modal analgesia and regional techniques to minimize opioid use.
  - There is also a recommendation to place sucrose/dextrose on the tongue to reduce pain during naso/orogastric tube placement in children.
  - ERAS also suggests to restart enteral feeds within the next 24–48 h after surgery, including breast-feeding, irrespective of the status of bowel function. Breast feeding is proven to be as effective and comforting as various analgesics in infants [28–31].

10.1.7 Non-pharmacological Methods of Pain Management in Children

1. *Distraction Techniques:* Methods such as reading fairy tales, playing cartoons or movies, or offering toys, playing video games help divert the child's attention from their pain, offering psychological comfort alongside analgesia.
2. *Virtual Reality (VR) and Augmented Reality (AR):* Recently, use of goggles and VR headsets to simulate an immersive 3D world are being used to manage emotional and psychological aspect of pain during venous cannulation, pediatric dental pro-

cedures, and wound dressing for burns. VR games can be used to counter anxiety experienced by children on entering unfamiliar environment of an operation theatre [32–34].

10.1.7.1 Routes of Analgesic Administration

The route should be as comfortable as possible for the child. Intravenous (IV) and oral routes are preferred, but if these are not feasible, other routes such as rectal, nasal, or transmucosal may be considered.

1. *Intravenous Analgesia:* Commonly used in pediatric patients, either in single doses or continuous infusions, especially in Pediatric Intensive Care Units (PICUs). Options include:
   - *PCA (Patient-Controlled Analgesia):* Children may self-administer a preset dose of analgesics.
   - *NCA (Nurse-Controlled Analgesia):* For younger or cognitively impaired children.
2. *Subcutaneous Administration*: Recommended for oncological or hospice patients (e.g., morphine). Transdermal patches can also be used in some cases.
3. *Rectal Administration:* This method is acceptable if oral or IV routes are not feasible, but it should be avoided in immunosuppressed children due to the risk of perianal abscesses.
4. *Nasal and Transmucosal Routes:* These alternatives, particularly nasal opioid administration (e.g., fentanyl, sufentanil, ketamine), are attractive for situations where IV access is not possible, such as burns or home care. However, these options may not always be approved for pediatric use in certain regions.
5. *Regional Anesthesia:* Regional anesthesia techniques can be valuable in pediatric pain management, where feasible. Administering local anesthetics (LA) into the surgical wound before or during surgery significantly complements perioperative pain control [35–39].

10.1.8 Pharmacotherapy of Pain in Children

10.1.8.1 Opioid Analgesics

- Opioids are widely used in pediatric pain management, especially for moderate to severe pain.
- *Mechanism*: *Mu opioid receptor agonists,* which relieve pain but also affect mood, behavior, and various bodily functions, such as respiration and digestion.
- *Routes of Administration.*
  - *Intravenous (IV)* is the most common route for opioids in perioperative care. Alternatives like *subcutaneous, oral, or transdermal* routes offer flexibility for specific clinical needs.
  - *Continuous infusion or Patient-Controlled Analgesia (PCA)* is typically used in PICUs to provide sustained pain relief, especially for severe pain.
  - *Combination therapy:* To reduce the total opioid dose and side effects, opioids are often combined with other analgesics.
- *Specific Opioids.*
  1. *Morphine*: A gold standard opioid, its pharmacokinetics in children resemble those in adults but require dose adjustments for premature infants and neonates due to immature organs. Dose 25–100 μg/kg.
  2. *Fentanyl*: 100 times more potent than morphine with a short half-life of 20–30 min, it is being used to manage acute pain perioperatively. Dose 1–2 μg/kg.
  3. *Sufentanil:* 1000 times more potent than morphine, it is restricted to PICUs due to its potency and risks. Dose 0.5–1 μg/kg bolus followed by continuous infusion of 0.5 to 1 μg/kg/h.
  4. *Oxycodone:* Effective for children over 12 years old, available in both oral and IV forms, making it useful for sequential therapy as children transition from IV to oral analgesics.

5. *Tramadol:* A weak opioid that also inhibits norepinephrine reuptake and increases serotonin release, it has faced restrictions in pediatric use. The FDA forbade its use in children due to safety concerns, but the European Society for Pediatric Anesthesiologists still allows its hospital-based use in Europe. However, interactions like exacerbation of postoperative nausea with ondansetron should be avoided.

- *Agonist/Antagonist Drugs*
  Medications, such as *Nalbuphine*, have a ceiling effect that limits respiratory depression but also limits efficacy at higher doses. Nalbuphine is often used for mild to moderate postoperative pain and can be combined with morphine for enhanced pain control.
- *Side Effects*
  - Common side effects include nausea, vomiting, constipation, sedation, and the serious risk of respiratory depression.
  - Concerns like *opioid-induced hyperalgesia*, where increasing doses paradoxically worsen pain, and increased tolerance have been noted with short-acting opioids.
  - *Immunosuppression:* Most opioids can cause immunosuppression, increasing the risk of postoperative infections.
  - *Opioid-induced Hyperalgesia (OIH):* Ultra-short-acting opioids, such as remifentanil, may paradoxically increase pain despite higher opioid doses [35–39].

10.1.8.2 Non-opioid Analgesics

This topic is discussed at length in a separate chapter on "Methods of Analgesia," however for sake of completion of chapter, we have mentioned it here. In the pediatric age group, the key differences in the use of non-opioid analgesics pertain to dosage adjustments, route of administration, and specific considerations regarding their pharmacokinetics and adverse effects.

1. *Paracetamol*
   - Dosage:
     - Intravenous: Loading dose remains 15–20 mg/kg, followed by maintenance doses (10–15 mg/kg every 6–8 h). Maximum cumulative daily dose must be tailored to weight and age, especially in neonates and infants with immature liver enzymes.
     - Oral: 10–15 mg/kg per dose; maximum total daily dose is 60 mg/kg/day in most pediatric populations but may be adjusted for premature neonates due to slower metabolism.
     - Rectal: Higher doses (20–40 mg/kg) are necessary due to variable bioavailability, with reduced dosing (15 mg/kg) for infants <10 kg.
   - Specific Considerations
     - Neonates have reduced metabolic capacity; dosing frequency may need adjustment.
     - Risk of hepatotoxicity increases in malnourished children or those with liver dysfunction.
     - Monitoring is crucial to prevent cumulative overdose in febrile illnesses.
2. Metamizole
   - Dosage:
     - Short-term continuous infusion: Pediatric dose is 2.5 mg/kg/hour for effective analgesia.
     - Intermittent dosing: 10–15 mg/kg every 8 hours.
   - Specific Considerations:
     - Hypotension: This is a notable concern in children during rapid intravenous administration. Dosing must be done slowly and with hemodynamic monitoring.
     - *Risk of agranulocytosis*: This remains a rare but severe side effect, requiring careful consideration for repeated or prolonged use.
3. *NSAIDs*
   - *Dosage of commonly used NSAIDs:*
   - *Ibuprofen*: Oral, rectal, and intravenous doses remain 10 mg/kg every 8 h.

- *Diclofenac*: Oral: 1 mg/kg 8 hourly. Rectal: 0.5–1 mg/kg 8 hourly.
- *Ketorolac*: Intravenous: 0.5–1 mg/kg as a single dose, then 0.15–0.2 mg/kg every 6 h (maximum single dose: 30 mg; maximum maintenance dose: 10 mg).
- *Ketoprofen*: Intravenous: 1 mg/kg every 8 h.
- Specific Considerations:
  - Hypotension: This is a notable concern in children during rapid intravenous administration. Dosing must be done slowly and with hemodynamic monitoring.
  - Risk of agranulocytosis: This remains a rare but severe side effect, requiring careful consideration for repeated or prolonged use [39–41].

10.1.8.3 Non-opioid Adjuvants

Non opioid adjuvants are used to enhance pain relief and manage side effects caused by other analgesics.

1. *Gabapentinoids*
   - *Gabapentin* and *pregabalin* are used to manage chronic neuropathic pain in children, though their use is off-label.
   - These drugs are incorporated into multimodal analgesia during the perioperative period, improving the quality of analgesia and reducing opioid requirements.
   - *Side effects* like nausea, vomiting, and urine retention are reduced with these drugs.
   - *Dose*: Gabapentin can be dosed at 10 mg/kg in younger children or 300 mg for children above 12 years.
   - The safety of pregabalin in children under 17 years has not been established.
2. *Alpha-2 Adrenergic Receptor Agonists*
   - *Clonidine* and *dexmedetomidine* are commonly used in perioperative pain management by inhibiting pain transmission at the *spinal cord and supraspinal level.*
   - These drugs help reduce postoperative opioid needs and the incidence of nausea, but they can cause *hypotension, bradycardia, and sedation.*

- Dexmedetomidine is typically used in doses ranging from 0.3 to 1 μg/kg intravenously, either as a single bolus or continuous infusion.
- Clonidine and dexmedetomidine are also being used as effective adjuncts in spinal, epidural, caudal blocks in children.

3. *Ketamine*
   - Ketamine is an NMDA receptor antagonist that provides analgesia, prevents persistent postoperative pain, and supports hemodynamic stability in patients.
   - It is effective in sub-anesthetic doses for perioperative analgesia without causing respiratory depression.
   - *Dose*: Doses typically range from 0.1 to 0.3 mg/kg for bolus administration, and continuous infusion doses are 0.06 to 0.12 mg/kg/h.
   - Preservative free Ketamine is also being used as an adjunct in peripheral nerve blocks and caudal blocks.
4. *Corticosteroids*
   - *Dexamethasone* is used for its anti-inflammatory and anti-nociceptive properties, especially in head and neck surgeries and procedures lasting longer than an hour.
   - It reduces pain intensity, opioid requirements, and postoperative nausea and vomiting.
   - A single dose of dexamethasone (0.1–0.5 mg/kg) has demonstrated no effect on increasing infection rates or delaying wound healing.
5. *Magnesium Sulfate*
   - Magnesium acts as an NMDA receptor antagonist and has anti-inflammatory properties, though evidence supporting its use in postoperative pain management in children is limited.
   - Doses typically involve a 30–50 mg/kg bolus followed by a continuous infusion of 15 mg/kg/h.
   - Magnesium can delay neuromuscular conduction and cause bradycardia [42–44].

10.1.9 Regional Analgesia in Children

Regional anesthesia provides superior and prolonged pain control compared to systemic analgesia, reducing the need for opioids. Peripheral nerve blocks in children are similar to those in adults, but require adaptations due to smaller anatomical structures. Common landmark guided blocks being given by pediatric anesthesiologists are bilateral infraorbital nerve block for cleft lip and palate surgery; caudal block for hip, anal, perineal, or abdominal surgeries; penile block in hypospadias repair; femoral block; fascia iliaca block, etc. Many upper and lower extremity blocks are being given using nerve stimulators alone, or combined with landmark technique. Ultrasound guidance improves the safety and efficacy of regional blocks. Regional blocks in children should always be performed under general anesthesia or deep sedation. Test doses of local anesthetics, monitoring for acute compartment syndrome, and managing toxic complications like local anesthetic systemic toxicity (LAST) are crucial considerations.

Newer regional anesthesia techniques being performed using ultrasound in children are:

1. *Quadratus Lumborum (QL) Block:* Provides effective analgesia for thoracoabdominal and lower abdominal surgeries, such as appendectomy or hernia repair, under ultrasound guidance.
2. *Erector Spinae Pain (ESP) Block:* ESP block is being utilized for pain relief in including thoracotomies, rib fractures, or laparoscopic procedures.
3. *Suprainguinal fascia iliaca (FI) block*: Widely used for pain relief in orthopedic procedures involving the hip or knee, such as femur fractures or hip osteotomies. [43–45]

10.2 Special Considerations in Pediatric Pain Management

10.2.1 Acute Post-traumatic Pain in Emergency Room

- *Pain Mechanism:* Acute post-traumatic pain is mixed, involving nociceptive and neuropathic components, with a dominant inflammatory response due to tissue damage.
- *Pain Management:* Play and distraction techniques help the child cope with the injury, bleeding and the anxiety of being in an unfamiliar environment. Soothing presence of a parent or trusted guardian while application of splints and dressings can help. Proper pain intensity assessment, using the various tools mentioned, is crucial for effective management as follows:
  - *Mild Pain (VAS/NRS/FlACC 1–3):* For milder pain, Paracetamol 20 mg/kg loading dose followed by 15 mg/kg 4–6 hourly can be administered orally or rectally. NSAIDS like Oral Ibuprofen 10 mg/kg 6–8 hourly may also be given.
  - *Moderate Pain (VAS/NRS/FlACC 4–6):* Paracetamol in the above-mentioned dose along with NSAIDS like Tab Diclofenac 1 mg/kg 8 hourly or Tab ibuprofen 10 mg/kg 6–8 hourly can be given. If needed, opioids like Oral Codeine 1 mg/kg 4–6 hourly (for age >12 years) or Oral morphine 0.2–0.5 mg/kg stat can be used as a rescue measure.
  - *Severe Pain (VAS/NRS/FlACC >7):* Entonox can be used as a holding measure to calm down the child until intravenous cannulation is established and stronger opioids like intranasal diamorphine (0.1 mg/kg) or intravenous morphine (0.1–0.2 mg/kg) can be administered. Fentanyl (1.5 mcg/kg) is a potent opioid but should be used cautiously as it comes with a high risk of muscle rigidity (thoracic/glottic) and respiratory failure, particularly in non-intubated children. Ketamine (100–300 mcg/kg) can be useful in cases where pain persists despite NSAIDS and opioids. Antiemetics like Ondansetron should be used liberally to manage nausea arising from use of opioids [46, 47].

10.3 Conclusion

Effective pediatric pain management is crucial to ensure the well-being and comfort of children undergoing surgical procedures or suffering from acute or chronic pain. A comprehensive approach, which includes thorough assessment, appropriate pharmacological interventions, and non-pharmacological strategies, is essential for achieving optimal outcomes. It is important to recognize that pediatric pain is often underreported and undertreated, which necessitates the involvement of a multidisciplinary team and family-centered care.

References

1. Mak WY, Yuen V, Irwin M, Hui T. Pharmacotherapy for acute pain in children: current practice and recent advances. Expert Opin Pharmacother. 2011;12(6):865–81. https://doi.org/10.1517/14656566.2011.542751. Epub 2011 Jan 22. PMID: 21254863.
2. Eccleston C, Fisher E, Howard RF, Slater R, Forgeron P, Palermo TM, et al. Delivering transformative action in paediatric pain: a Lancet Child & Adolescent Health Commission. Lancet Child Adolesc Health. 2021;5(1):47–87. https://doi.org/10.1016/S2352-4642(20)30277-7.
3. Krauss BS, Calligaris L, Green SM, Barbi E. Current concepts in management of pain in children in the emergency department. Lancet. 2016;387(10013):83–92. https://doi.org/10.1016/S0140-6736(14)61686-X.
4. Groenewald CB, Rabbitts JA, Schroeder DR, Harrison TE. Prevalence of moderate to severe pain in hospitalized children. Pediatr Anesth. 2012;22:661–8.
5. Stewart DW, Ragg PG, Sheppard S, Chalkiadis GA. The severity and duration of postoperative pain and analgesia requirements in children after tonsillectomy, orchidopexy, or inguinal hernia repair. Paediatr Anaesth. 2012;22:136–43.
6. Stanko D, Bergesio R, Davies K, Hegarty M, von Ungern-Sternberg BS. Postoperative pain, nausea and vomiting following adeno-tonsillectomy–a long-term follow-up. Pediatr Anesth. 2013;23:690–6. https://doi.org/10.1111/pan.12170.
7. Nair S, Neil MJ. Paediatric pain: physiology, assessment and pharmacology. ATOTW. 2013;289:1–10. Dubin AE, Patapoutian A. Nociceptors: the sensors of the pain pathway. J Clin Investig 2010;120:3760–3772. 10.1172/JCI42843.

8. Djouhri L, Lawson SN. Abeta-fiber nociceptive primary afferent neurons: a review of incidence and properties in relation to other afferent A-fiber neurons in mammals. Brain Res Brain Res Rev. 2004;46(2):131–45. https://doi.org/10.1016/j.brainresrev.2004.07.015.
9. Zeltzer LK, Bush JP, Chen E, Riveral A. A psychobiologic approach to pediatric pain: part 1. History, physiology, and assessment strategies. Curr Probl Pediatr. 1997;27(6):225–53. https://doi.org/10.1016/s0045-9380(97)80025-4.
10. Garland EL. Pain processing in the human nervous system: a selective review of nociceptive and biobehavioral pathways. Prim Care. 2012;39(3):561–71. https://doi.org/10.1016/j.pop.2012.06.013.
11. Gaglani A, Gross T. Pediatric pain management. Emerg Med Clin North Am. 2018;36(2):323–34. https://doi.org/10.1016/j.emc.2017.12.002.
12. Cassidy RC, Walco GA. Pediatric pain: ethical issues and ethical management. Child Health Care. 1996;25(4):253–64.
13. Segerdahl M, Warren-Stomberg M, Rawal N, Brattwall M, Jakobsson J. Children in day surgery: clinical practice and routines. The results from a nation-wide survey. Acta Anaesthesiol Scand. 2008;52:821–8. https://doi.org/10.1111/j.1399-6576.2008.01669.
14. Walco GA, Burns JP, Cassidy RC. The ethics of pain control in infants and children. N Engl J Med. 1994;331(8):541–4.
15. Gehdoo RP. Post operative pain management in paediatric patients. Indian J Anaesth. 2004;48(5):406–14.
16. Wilson GA, Doyle E. Validation of three paediatric pain scores for use by parents. Anaesthesia. 1996;51(11):1005–7.
17. Zieliński J, Morawska KM, Zatoński T. Pain assessment and management in children in the postoperative period: a review of the most commonly used postoperative pain assessment tools, new diagnostic methods and the latest guidelines for postoperative pain therapy in children. Adv Clin Exp Med. 2020;29(365–74):365. https://doi.org/10.17219/acem/112600.
18. van Dijk M, de Boer JB, Koot HM, Tibboel D, Passchier J, Duivenvoorden HJ. The reliability and validity of the COMFORT scale as a postoperative pain instrument in 0 to 3-year-old infants. Pain. 2000;84:367–77. https://doi.org/10.1016/S0304-3959(99)00239-0.
19. Suraseranivongse S, Kaosaard R, Intakong P, Pornsiriprasert S, Karnchana Y, Kaopinpruck J, et al. A comparison of postoperative pain scales in neonates. Br J Anaesth. 2006;97(4):540–4. https://doi.org/10.1093/bja/ael184.
20. Shrestha-Ranjit JM, Manias E. Pain assessment and management practices in children following surgery of the lower limb. J Clin Nurs. 2010;19:118–28.
21. Taylor EM, Boyer K, Campbell FA. Pain in hospitalized children: a prospective cross-sectional survey of pain prevalence, intensity, assessment

and management in a Canadian pediatric teaching hospital. Pain Res Manag. 2008;13:25–32.
22. Holthusen H, Eichwede F, Stevens M, Willnow U, Lipfert P. Pre-emptive analgesia: comparison of preoperative with postoperative caudal block on postoperative pain in children. Br J Anaesth. 1994;73:440–2.
23. El-Fattah AM, Ramzy E. Pre-emptive triple analgesia protocol for tonsillectomy pain control in children: double-blind, randomised, controlled, clinical trial. J Laryngol Otol. 2013;127(4):383–91. https://doi.org/10.1017/S0022215113000364.
24. Martin LD, Jimenez N, Lynn AM. A review of perioperative anesthesia and analgesia for infants: updates and trends to watch. F1000Res. 2017;6(120):120. https://doi.org/10.12688/f1000research.10272.1.
25. Cettler M, Zielińska M, Rosada-Kurasińska J, Kubica-Cielińska A, Jarosz K, Bartkowska-Śniatkowska A. Guidelines for treatment of acute pain in children–the consensus statement of the Section of Paediatric Anaesthesiology and Intensive Therapy of the Polish Society of Anaesthesiology and Intensive Therapy. Anaesthesiol Intensive Ther. 2022;54:197–218.
26. Salekin MS, Mouton PR, Zamzmi G, Patel R, Goldgof D, Kneusel M, et al. Future roles of artificial intelligence in early pain management of newborns. Paediatr Neonatal Pain. 2021;3(3):134–45.
27. Rey R, Gualtieri R, La Scala G, Barbe KP. Artificial intelligence in the diagnosis and management of appendicitis in pediatric departments: a systematic review. Eur J Pediatr Surg. 2024;34:385.
28. Brindle ME, Heiss K, Scott MJ, Herndon CA, Ljungqvist O, Koyle MA. on behalf Pediatric ERAS (Enhanced Recovery After Surgery) Society. Embracing change: the era for pediatric ERAS is here. Pediatr Surg Int. 2019;35(6):631–4. https://doi.org/10.1007/s00383-019-04476-3.
29. Shinnick JK, Short HL, Heiss KF, Santore MT, Blakely ML, Raval MV. Enhancing recovery in pediatric surgery: a review of the literature. J Surg Res. 2016;202(1):165–76. https://doi.org/10.1016/j.jss.2015.12.051.
30. Gibb ACN, Crosby MA, McDiarmid C, Urban D, Lam JYK, Wales PW, et al. Creation of an Enhanced Recovery After Surgery (ERAS) Guideline for neonatal intestinal surgery patients: a knowledge synthesis and consensus generation approach and protocol study. BMJ Open. 2018;8(12):e023651. https://doi.org/10.1136/bmjopen-2018-023651.
31. Pearson KL, Hall NJ. What is the role of enhanced recovery after surgery in children? A scoping review. Pediatr Surg Int. 2017;33:42–51. https://doi.org/10.1007/s00383-016-3986.
32. Ibitoye MB, Dawson P. The effectiveness of distraction as procedural pain management technique in pediatric oncology patients: a meta-analysis and systematic review. JPSM. 2017;54:589–600. https://doi.org/10.1016/j.jpainsymman.2017.07.006.

33. Alqudimat M, Mesaroli G, Lalloo C, Stinson J, Matava C. State of the art: immersive technologies for perioperative anxiety, acute, and chronic pain management in pediatric patients. Curr Anesthesiol Rep. 2021;11(3):265–74. https://doi.org/10.1007/s40140-021-00472-3. Epub 2021 Jul 14. PMID: 34276254; PMCID: PMC8277426.
34. Ang SP, Montuori M, Trimba Y, Maldari N, Patel D, Chen QC. Recent applications of virtual reality for the management of pain in burn and pediatric patients. Curr Pain Headache Rep. 2021;25(1):4. https://doi.org/10.1007/s11916-020-00917-0.
35. Lönnqvist PA, Morton NS. Postoperative analgesia in infants and children. Br J Anaesth. 2005;95(1):59–68.
36. Kart T, Christrup LL, Rasmussen M. Recommended use of morphine in neonates, infants and children based on a literature review: part 1–pharmacokinetics. Paediatr Anaesth. 1997;7:5–11. https://doi.org/10.1046/j.1460-9592.1997.d01-30.x.
37. Rosen DM, Alcock MM, Palmer GM. Opioids for acute pain management in children. Anaesth Intensive Care. 2022;50(1–2):81–94.
38. Vittinghoff M, Lönnqvist PA, Mossetti V, Heschl S, Simic D, Colovic V, et al. Postoperative Pain Management in children: guidance from the Pain Committee of the European Society for Paediatric Anaesthesiology (ESPA Pain Management Ladder Initiative) Part II. Anaesth Crit Care Pain Med. 2024;43(6):101427. https://doi.org/10.1016/j.accpm.2024.101427. Epub 2024 Sep 17. PMID: 39299468.
39. Zhu A, Benzon HA, Anderson TA. Evidence for the efficacy of systemic opioid-sparing analgesics in pediatric surgical populations: a systematic review. Anesth Analg. 2017;125(5):1569–87.
40. Cooney MF. Pain management in children: NSAID use in the perioperative and emergency department settings. Paediatr Drugs. 2021;23(4):361–72. https://doi.org/10.1007/s40272-021-00449-z. Epub 2021 May 28. PMID: 34046854; PMCID: PMC8275553.
41. Kościelniak-Merak B, Batko I, Kobylarz K, Sztefko K, Tomasik PJ. Intravenous, perioperatively administered lidocaine regulates serum pain modulators' concentrations in children undergoing spinal surgery. Pain Med. 2020;21:1464–73. https://doi.org/10.1093/pm/pnz212.
42. Mayell A, Srinivasan I, Campbell F, Peliowski A. Analgesic effects of gabapentin after scoliosis surgery in children: a randomized controlled trial. Pediatr Anesth. 2014;24(12):1239–44.
43. Anderson BJ, Palmer GM. Recent pharmacological advances in paediatric analgesics. Biomed Pharmacother. 2006;60(7):303–9.
44. Suresh S, Schaldenbrand K, Wallis B, De Oliveira Jr GS. Regional anaesthesia to improve pain outcomes in paediatric surgical patients: a qualitative systematic review of randomized controlled trials. Br J Anaesth. 2014;113(3):375–90.

45. Walter CM, Abbasian N, Olbrecht VA. Trends in pediatric pain: thinking beyond opioids. Anesthesiol Clin. 2020;38(3):663–78. https://doi.org/10.1016/j.anclin.2020.04.002. Epub 2020 Jul 16. PMID: 32792190.
46. Häske D, Böttiger BW, Bouillon B, Fischer M, Gaier G, Gliwitzky B, et al. Analgesia in patients with trauma in emergency medicine: a systematic review and meta-analysis. Dtsch Arztebl Int. 2017;114(46):785.
47. Greenwald M. Analgesia for the pediatric trauma patient: primum non nocere? Clin Pediatr Emerg Med. 2010;11(1):28–40.

MIX
Papier aus verantwortungsvollen Quellen
Paper from responsible sources
FSC® C105338

If you have any concerns about our products,
you can contact us on
ProductSafety@springernature.com

In case Publisher is established outside the EU,
the EU authorized representative is:
Springer Nature Customer Service Center GmbH
Europaplatz 3, 69115 Heidelberg, Germany

Printed by Libri Plureos GmbH
in Hamburg, Germany